CURE

KIDNEY STONE *(Hasat-e-Kulliya)*

With Herbal Medicine

By

Dr Zaid Iqbal

MS (Ilmul Jarhat) NIUM

Assistant Professor

MTC Mansoora Malegaon

&

Dr. Abuzar Lari

MD (Ilaj-Bit-Tadbeer) NIUM

Assistant Professor

MTC Mansoora Malegaon

DEDICATED

TO

MY FATHER IQBAL AHMED

MY MOTHER RAZIYA BANO

&

MY TEACHERS AND FRIENDS

PREFACE

The practice of *Unani* medicine is based on the basic principles of *Akhlat* (humors), *Mizaj* (temperament), etc. which explain by eminent *Unani* physicians. In this book we tried to explain the concept of *Hasat-e-kulliya* (Renal stone), their causes, history taking, clinical examination, investigation, and the addition to detailed line of treatment in cases of renal stone. The firm foundation of *Unani* concept will help the physicians in arriving at a provisional diagnosis and for planning relevant necessary investigations to confirm the diagnosis. This book is dedicated to the community of medical students whose thirst for knowledge make the teachers learn. Learning helps in the proper management of patients. Medicine is an ever changing science. The vast clinical experience, the technological advancement in the field of investigatory modalities, tremendous explosion in the invention and addition of newer drugs in the field of pharmacology, and a wide variety of interventional therapeutic advancements have contributed to the voluminous growth of medical literature. Human brain cannot remember all the facts. It is impossible to learn, register, Remember and to recall all the medical facts in the course of time bound undergraduate and postgraduate medical education. It is the realization of these difficulties that prompted me to write this book. Hence, an earnest attempt has been made to merge the clinical methods and the principles of *Unani* medicine and to present both in a condensed form. To explain the *Unani* concept and literature about renal stone and its management along with surgical aspect was the main theme of this book. This book intended primarily for medical undergraduates and also for postgraduate hospital doctors, particularly those studying for higher clinical examinations or returning to clinical practice. The book is also an essential reference for *Unani* practitioners.

Dr Zaid Iqbal

ACKNOWLEGMENT

All praises be to "Almighty Allah" the lord of the world, the most beneficent and merciful and peace be upon his Prophet Mohammed (SAWS). Through the grace of Almighty Allah, the uphill task has been accomplished.

Foremost I would like to express my deep sense of gratitude to my beloved parents especially to my father *Mr. Iqbal Ahmad,* for their Support and Guidance. I pray to Allah to show mercy to them and forgive them. I greatly appreciate the constructive suggestions and help that we have received from past and present friends, colleagues and focus groups in the design and content of the book. I Thankfull to my Guide *Dr. Mohd Shakeel Ansari*, Lecturer, Dept. of Jarahat, National Institute of Unani Medicine, Bengaluru, for their collaboration.

I am thankfull to my teacher *Dr. Rashid Qazi Sir* Principal M.I.J Tibbiya Unani Medical College, Mumbai for their Guidance for post-graduation and unconditional moral support.

Also I would like to express my eternal and deep sense my friends, *Dr. Abuzar lari, Dr.Mussarat Ali, Dr.Ansari Mushir* and *Dr.Shahzad sr.* I always obliged to him for his support and cooperation, and their suggestion.

INDEX

HASAT -E- KULLIYA   (KIDNEY STONE)   حصات كلية

Surgical physiology & Anatomy of Urinary system

(Kidney, ureter and urinary bladder):

The urinary system's function is to filter blood and create urine as a waste by-product. The organs of the urinary system include the kidneys, renal pelvis, ureters, bladder and urethra. The body takes nutrients from food and converts them to energy. After the body has taken the food components that it needs, waste products are left behind in the bowel and in the blood. The kidney and urinary systems help the body to eliminate liquid waste called urea, and to keep chemicals, such as potassium, sodium, and water in balance. Urea is produced when foods containing protein, such as meat, poultry, and certain vegetables, are broken down in the body. Urea is carried in the bloodstream to the kidneys, where it is removed along with water and other wastes in the form of urine.

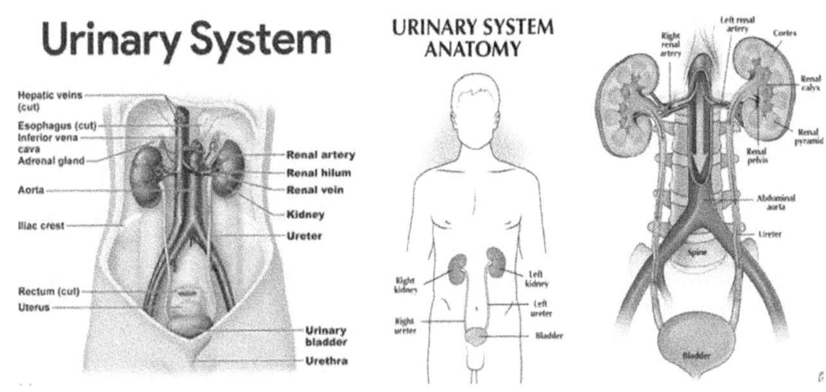

Kidney

Synonyms: Nephros, Renes, *Kulliya, Gurda*

Kidney excrete end product of metabolism and excess water. These actions are essential for control of concentration of various substance in the body maintaining electrolyte and water balance approximately constant in tissue fluid.

Kidney also have endocrine function producing and releasing erythropoietin which affects red blood cell formation, renin; which influence blood pressure, 1,25-dihydroxycholecalciferole which is involved in the control of calcium absorption, mineral metabolism and various other soluble factors with metabolic action.

- ➤ Kidneys are pair of vital excretory organ situated in posterior abdominal wall, behind the peritoneum, one on each side of vertebral column.
- ➤ They remove waste product of metabolism and excess of water and salts from the blood and maintain its PH.
- ➤ It maintains water & electrolyte balance by excreting hydrogen ion and bicarbonate ion.
- ➤ It maintain acid base balance by excreting hydrogen ion and bicarbonate ion.
- ➤ It forms erythropoietin which is must for normal erythropoiesis.
- ➤ It secretes renin. Renin is an enzyme with vasoconstrictor effect. Increased renin production results in HTN.
- ➤ Metabolism of Vit D.
- ➤ Size: Each kidney is approximately (11x3x6cm) 11cm long, 6cm broad, 3cm thick.
- ➤ Weight: 150gms in Male and 135gms in Female.
- ➤ Colour: Reddish brown.
- ➤ Shape: Bean shaped.
- ➤ Kidneys occupy the epigastric, hypochondric, lumbar and umbilical regions.
- ➤ Vertically they extend from the upper border of 12th thoracic vertebrae to centre of the body of 3rd lumbar vertebrae.
- ➤ Because of Liver the right kidney is slightly lower than the left, and the left kidney is a little nearer to the median plane then the right.
- ➤ Left kidney is nearer to vertebral column as compared to right.
- ➤ The transpyloric plane passes through the upper part of the hilus of the right kidney and through the lower part of the hilus of the left kidney.
- ➤ Long axis of the kidney is directed downwards and laterally, so that the upper poles are nearer to median plane than the lower poles. The transverse axis is directed laterally and backwards.
- ➤ Approximate distance of kidney from midline is about 5cm.
- ➤ In the foetus kidney is lobulated and is made up of about 12 lobules. After birth the lobules gradually fuse, so that in adults the kidney is uniformly smooth.
- ➤ Each kidney is bean shaped. It has upper and lower poles, medial and lateral borders, and anterior and posterior surfaces.

> Lower pole is palpable in Lin and thin person at renal angle.

> Both kidneys moves 2cm up and down with respiration.

> Kidney is abdominal organ but embryologically it develops as a pelvic organ and initially its position vary. It is non rotated means its hilum faces anteriorly. Ascend from pelvic to abdomen and rotation of kidney takes place in between 5-8 weeks of foetal life. As kidney ascends, it comes to its normal abdominal position and as undergoes in medial rotation so that hilum which initially faced anteriorly, now after rotation faced medially towards the vertebral column.

<u>Applied surgical anatomy</u>:

Hilum

The following structures are seen in the hilum from anterior side to posterior side.

- The renal vein
- The renal artery
- The renal pelvis, which is the expanded upper end of the ureter.

Examination of these structures enables the anterior and posterior aspects of the kidney to be distinguished from each other. As the pelvis is continuous inferiorly with the ureter, the superior and inferior poles of the kidney can also be distinguished by examining the hilum. So it is possible to determine the side to which a kidney belongs by examining the structures in the hilum. Commonly, one of the branches of the renal artery enters the hilus behind the renal pelvis, and a tributary of the renal vein may be found in the same plane.

RELATIONS OF THE KIDNEYS

The kidneys are retroperitoneal organs and are only partly covered by peritoneum anteriorly.

<u>Relations Common to the Two Kidneys</u>

1. The upper pole of each kidney is related to the corresponding suprarenal gland. The lower poles lie about 2.5 cm above the iliac crests.

2. The medial border of each kidney is related to:

a. The suprarenal gland, above the hilus, and

b. To the ureter below the hilus.

3. Posterior relations: The posterior surfaces of both kidneys are related to the following.

a. Diaphragm

b. Medial and lateral arcuate ligaments

c. Psoas major

d. Quadratus lumborum

e. Transversus abdominis

f. Subcostal vessels

g. Subcostal, iliohypogastric and ilioinguinal nerves.

In addition, the right kidney is related to twelfth rib, and the left kidney to eleventh and twelfth ribs.

4. The structures related to the hilum have been described earlier.

<u>Other Relations of the Right Kidney</u>

<u>Anterior Relations</u>

- Right suprarenal gland
- Liver
- Second part of duodenum
- Hepatic flexure of colon
- Small intestine

Out of these, the hepatic and intestinal surfaces are covered by peritoneum.

The lateral border of the right kidney is related to the right lobe of the liver and to the hepatic flexure of the colon.

<u>Other Relations of the Left Kidney</u>

<u>Anterior Relations</u>

- Left suprarenal gland
- Spleen

- Stomach
- Pancreas
- Splenic vessels
- Splenic flexure and descending colon
- Jejunum

Out of these, the gastric, splenic and jejunal surfaces are covered by peritoneum.

The lateral border of the left kidney is related to the spleen and to the descending colon.

CAPSULES OR COVERINGS OF KIDNEY

The Fibrous Capsule

This is a thin membrane which closely invests the kidney and lines the renal sinus. Normally, it can be easily stripped off from the kidney, but in certain diseases, it becomes adherent and cannot be stripped.

Perirenal or Perinephric Fat

This is a layer of adipose tissue lying outside the fibrous capsule. It is thickest at the borders of the kidney and fills up the extra space in the renal sinus.

Renal Fascia

The perirenal fascia was originally described as being made up of two separate layers.

Posterior layer was called fascia of Zuckerkandal and anterior layer as fascia of Gerota. These two fasciae fused laterally to form lateral conal fascia. According to this view, lateral conal fascia continued anterolaterally behind colon to blend with parietal peritoneum.

Pararenal or Paranephric Body (Fat)

It consists of a variable amount of fat lying outside the renal fascia. It is more abundant posteriorly and towards the lower pole of the kidney. It fills up the paravertebral gutter and forms a cushion for the kidney.

STRUCTURE

Naked eye examination of a coronal section of the kidney shows:

1. An outer—reddish brown cortex.

2. An inner—pale medulla.

3. A space—the renal sinus.

The renal medulla is made up of about 10 conical masses, called the renal pyramids. Their apices form the renal papillae which indent the minor calyces

VASCULAR SEGMENTS

The renal artery gives 5 segmental branches, 4 from its anterior division and one from its posterior division. The segments are apical, upper, middle and lower on anterior aspect. On posterior aspect, segments seen are posterior and parts of apical and lower segments.

The lymphatics of the kidney drain into the lateral aortic nodes located at the level of origin of the renal arteries (L2).

Nerve Supply The kidney is supplied by the renal plexus, an off shoot of the coeliac plexus. It contains sympathetic (T10–L1) fibres which are chiefly vasomotor. The afferent nerves of the kidney belong to segments T10 to T12.

EXPOSURE OF THE KIDNEY FROM BEHIND

In exposing the kidney from behind, the following layers have to be reflected one by one.

1. Skin

2. Superficial fascia

3. Posterior layer of thoracolumbar (lumbar) fascia with latissimus dorsi and serratus posterior inferior

4. Erector spinae, which can be removed for convenience

5. Middle layer of thoracolumbar fascia

6. Quadratus lumborum

7. Anterior layer of thoracolumbar fascia in which the related nerves are embedded.

Kidney pain especially kidney stone pain is referred at renal angle.

Any operation in case of kidney disease, lumbar incision is taken at renal angle.

Renal angle

Angle between lower border of 12th rib and outer border of erector spine muscles.

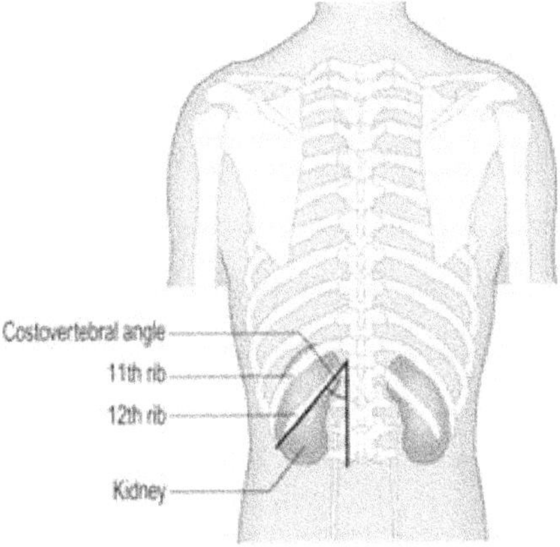

Ureter

Ureters are pair of muscular tubes which are attached proximally to the pelvis of kidney and distally to the bladder.

They are pair of narrow, thick walled muscular tubes which convey urine from the kidneys to the urinary bladder. They lie deep to the peritoneum, closely applied to the posterior abdominal wall in the upper part, and to the lateral pelvic wall in the lower part.

Each ureter is about 25cm (10 inches) long, of which the upper half (5 inches) lies in the abdomen, and the lower half (5 inches) in the pelvis. It measures about 3mm in diameter, but it is slightly constricted at five places.

It has abdominal and pelvic part. In its normal course, it has three parts:

1. Abdominal part
2. Pelvic part
3. Intravesical or intramural part.

Removal of stone from each of the above part of ureter by open surgery requires different surgical incision.

Ureter develops from part of ureteric bud that lies between pelvis of kidney and vesico-urethral canal.

Course: the ureter begins within the renal sinus as a funnel shaped dilatation, called the renal pelvis. The pelvis issues from the hilus of the kidney, descending along its medial margin or partly behind it. Gradually it narrows till the lower end of the kidney where it becomes the ureter proper.

The ureter passes downwards and slightly medially on the tips of transverse processes and the psoas major muscle, and enters the pelvis by crossing in front of termination of common iliac artery.

In the lesser or true pelvis the ureter at first runs downwards and slightly backwards and laterally, following the anterior margin of greater sciatic notch. Opposite the ischial spine it turns forward and medially to reach the base of the urinary bladder.

Normal Constrictions:

The ureter is slightly constricted at 5 places.

1. At the pelviuretric junction.
2. At the brim of lesser pelvic.
3. Point of crossing of ureter by ductus deference or broad ligament of uterus.
4. During its oblique passage through the bladder wall.
5. At its opening in lateral angle of trigone.

Ureter propels urine forward from pelvis of kidney into urinary bladder by the way of peristaltic waves. The urine cannot come back normally from bladder into ureter as ureteric orifices remains closed and does not allow back flow while bladder gets contracted for voiding of urine. This prevents ascend of infection from lower to upper urinary tract.

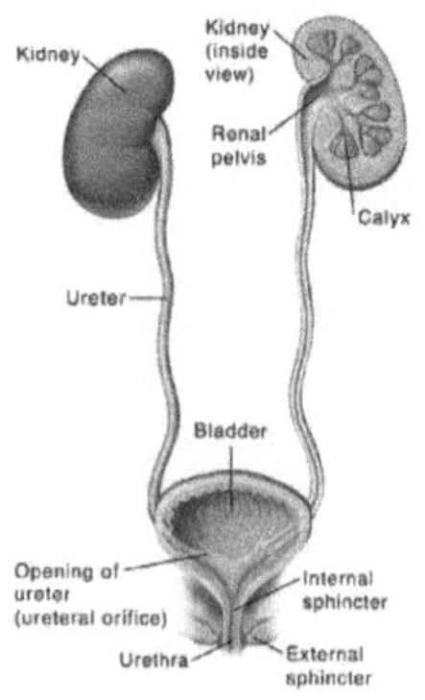

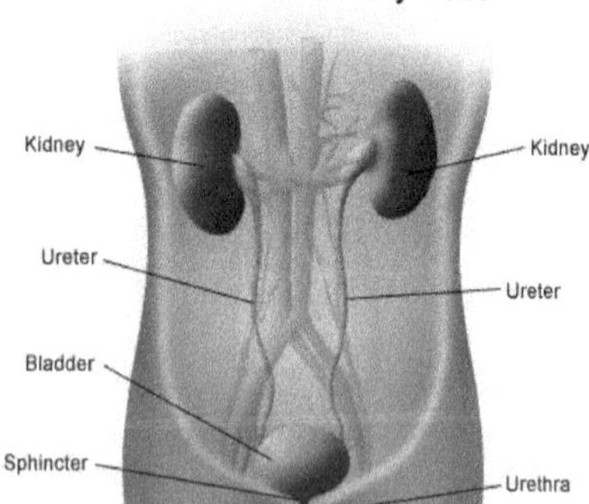

FIG: Urinary system

Urinary Bladder

The urinary bladder is a muscular sac in the pelvis, just above and behind the pubic bone. When empty, the bladder is about the size and shape of a pear.

Bladder is triangle-shaped, hollow organ is located in the lower abdomen. It is held in place by ligaments that are attached to other organs and the pelvic bones. The bladder's walls relax and expand to store urine, and contract and flatten to empty urine through the urethra. The typical healthy adult bladder can store up to two cups of urine for two to five hours.

Urinary bladder is temporary store house of urine which gets emptied through the urethra. The external urethral sphincter is the sphincter uretherae which is placed proximally in the wall of urethera, and not the terminal part of urethera. In case of pylorus and anal canal, the sphincters are placed at their terminal ends.

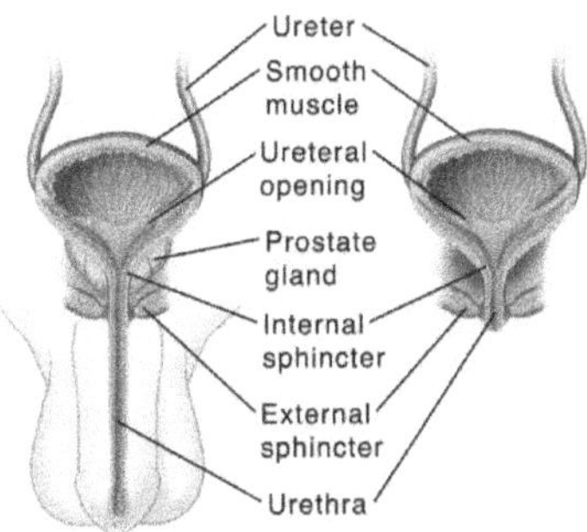

Urine is made in the kidneys and travels down two tubes called ureters to the bladder. The bladder stores urine, allowing urination to be infrequent and controlled. The bladder is lined by layers of muscle tissue that stretch to hold urine. The normal capacity of the bladder is 400-600 ml.

Capacity of the Bladder

The mean capacity of the bladder in an adult male is 220 ml, varying from 120 to 320 ml. Filling beyond 220 ml causes a desire to micturate, and the bladder is usually emptied when filled to about 250 to 300 ml. Filling up to 500 ml may be tolerated, but beyond this, it becomes painful. Referred pain is felt in the lower part of the anterior abdominal wall, perineum and penis (T11 to L2; S2 to S4).

During urination, the bladder muscles squeeze, and two sphincters (valves) open to allow urine to flow out. Urine exits the bladder into the urethra, which carries urine out of the body. Because it passes through the penis, the urethra is longer in men (8 inches) than in women (1.5 inches).

Upon examination, specific "landmarks" are used to describe the location of any irregularities in the bladder. These are:

Trigone: triangle-shaped region near the junction of the urethra & the bladder

Right and left lateral walls: walls on either side of the trigone

Posterior wall: back wall

Dome: roof of the bladder

- **Two sphincter muscles.** These circular muscles help keep urine from leaking by closing tightly like a rubber band around the opening of the bladder.

- **Nerves in the bladder.** The nerves alert a person when it is time to urinate, or empty the bladder.

Urethra

This tube allows urine to pass outside the body. The brain signals the bladder muscles to tighten, which squeezes urine out of the bladder. At the same time, the brain signals the sphincter muscles to relax to let urine exit the bladder through the urethra. When all the signals occur in the correct order, normal urination occurs.

The male urethra sub serving the function of urination and ejaculation, i.e expulsion of semen so it is 18-20cm long with curvatures and comprises preprostatic, prostatic, membranous, and longest anterior bulbar and penile parts.

The female urethra is for urination only and is 4cm long. The catheterisation if required is much easier in the female than in the male.

Facts about urine

- Normal, healthy urine is a pale straw or transparent yellow color.

- Darker yellow or honey colored urine means you need more water.
- A darker, brownish color may indicate a liver problem or severe dehydration.
- Pinkish or red urine may mean blood in the urine.

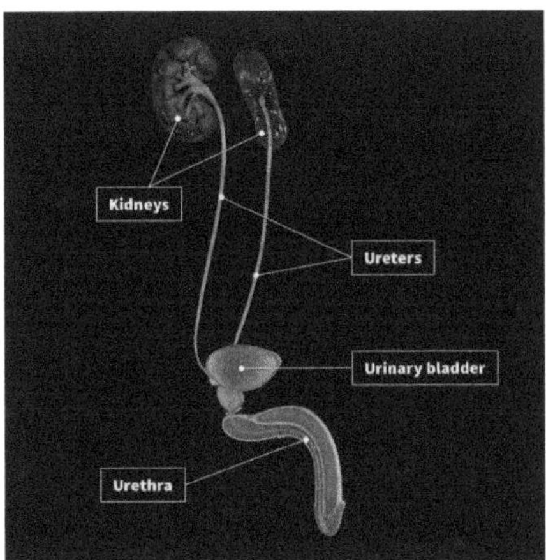

INTRODUCTION

Renal stone/ Kidney stone/ Urolithiasis

Kidney stones or Renal Calculi (from Latin renes, "kidney" and calculi, "pebbles") are solid structures composed of urinary precipitates and crystals. These stones can range in size from less than a millimetres to few centimetres. The word 'Crystal' is derived from the Greek word 'krystallosus' which means 'ice' and is used to refer to the solid phase of substances having a specific internal structure and enclosed by symmetrically arranged planner surface. Nephrolithiasis—from the Greek word nephros, meaning "kidney" and lithos, meaning "stone"—refers to the condition of having stones in the kidney or collecting system.

Urolithiasis (UL) is one of the most common diseases, with approximately 750 000 cases per year in Germany. Although most patients have only one stone episode, 25% of patients experience recurrent stone formation. UL therefore has a significant impact on quality of life and socioeconomic factors. The pathogenesis of calcium oxalate (CaOx), which accounts for >80% of all stones, is only incompletely understood.

The stone is a calculus of mineral or organic solids that can form anywhere in the urinary tract. In urinary tract stone is known as urolithiasis. Specifically when it present in the ureter termed as ureterolithiasis. As the stone passes through the urinary tract without causing any effect, it can be eliminated uneventfully (asymptomatic crystalluria) or can obstruct urinary flow, causing "colicky" pain as it passes. Renal colic is defined as severe intermittent flank pain that radiates to the groin, lower abdomen, or genitalia due to the passage of a stone through the urinary system. Pain is often accompanied by nausea, vomiting, dysuria and haematuria.

Renal stone disease has been recognized in many parts of the world since ancient era. It is one of the most painful and commonest urological disease. The evidence of urinary calculi has been found in 7000 years old Egyptian mummy. Its incidence has increased considerably during the 20th century. India is included in the stone belt region, consistently high incidence of Urolithiasis has been reported. It is estimated that at least 10% of the population in the industrialized part of the world is afflicted by urinary tract stone disease. Kidney stones are common in industrialized nations with an annual incidence of 0.5% to 1.9 %. In India upper and lower urinary tract stones occur frequently but the incidence shows wide regional variation. A high and progressively increasing incidence of urolithiasis has been reported in Udaipur and some other parts of Rajasthan in the western part of India. The commonest type of stones contains calcium in combination with either oxalate or phosphate. Calcium oxalate and calcium phosphate make up at least 80% of all kidney stones.

Infectious stones are composed of struvite or carbonate apatite crystals. Stones due to urinary tract infection make up approximately 15% of urinary stone diseases. Stones associated with infections are not only infectious stones but also other kinds of stones such as calcium oxalate. So any type of stone may become infected, but the term 'infectious stones' means that stone formation exclusively depends on Urea producing bacteria. Non- Urea producing bacteria may also be responsible for the synthesis of infectious stones. Uric acid, cystine and mixed type of stones make up rest of the urinary stones.

Normally urine has presence of organic and inorganic substances which inhibit crystallization of elements which leads to stone formation. Saturation is the point at which the water and the minerals dissolved in the urine are in equilibrium and precipitation does not occur below this level. Further increase in solute load leads to super saturation. It precipitates crystalline component which forms stone. Solute load is important, urine is complex solution so other factors influence saturation.

The strangest aspect of the history of urolithiasis is a relatively recent change in its epidemiology. Bladder stones were much more common than kidney stones until about 100 years ago and especially common in children. From last 70 years bladder stones have become very rare in children. During the last 30-40 years, urolithiasis has generally increased in human being. This increase has been blamed on increased protein diet. Other factors such as low fibre and excess of refined carbohydrate may predispose to urolithiasis. In particular, there may be peaks of increased urinary calcium following ingestion of sugary food or drinks. This, as part of the multifactorial problem of urolithiasis. In producing the renal stone, these mutually dependent elements are helped first of all by an overloaded stomach. Not least, perhaps, because of any increase in osmolarity and urine pH following digestion.

Factors affecting stone formation most important are urine output, the concentration of specific constituents, urine pH, and infection or damage within the urinary tract. It remains difficult, ultimately, to define why some individuals have stones and others do not. Attempts to analyse the relevant physical chemistry have overemphasized the behaviour of simple solutions. Urine is not a simple solution, many of its constituents are unknown and the ionic activity, as opposed to the total concentration, of many of the known solutes is still almost impossible to measure. For example, the presence of Tamm Hors fall protein increases crystal formation but only in whole urine and only at concentrations above 1300 mOsmI. Assessment of risk therefore needs to depend on measurement of ease of crystallization rather than composition.

In Unani system of Medicine the renal calculus is named as "*Hasat-e-Kulliya*" (Kidney stone), "*Hasat-e-Halib*" (Ureteric stone), "*Hasat-e-Masana*" (Bladder stone).

Ancient literatures described broadly the pathology, manifestations and treatment of *Hasat-e-kulliya*.

According to **Ali Ibne Abbas Majoosi**, renal calculi is formed due to increased *hararate ghareezia* of kidney and *Ghaleez madda* (viscid matter). The madda of these calculi derived from viscous humour (*khilt-e- ghaleez*) & mucous matter, these matters may be the *phlegmatic* or viscous blood or pus. Due to excessive *hararat* the *rutoobat* of this *ghaleez madda* is dried which after a period of time causes formation of stone. With these if there is constriction in passage of urine or ureter (*tang- e-majari*) causes the accumulation of small crystals and further it forms stone.

Sign and symptoms of renal stone is frequency and burning micturation with small crest (*reeg*) in the urine. Patients also having pain in flank region at the site of kidney which is sometime throbbing in nature. Patient also having complaint of pain at coccyx region and leg of affected side.

Rhazi mentioned the symptoms of calculi as renal pain, incontinence of urine, dysuria. The persons passing sandy precipitate in their urine must have the calculus in his kidneys or in urinary bladder. According to Rhazi when patient having dysuria with severe pain in flank and lower abdomen, with these patient having nausea and constipation, it indicate the stone in both kidney. Patient feeling heaviness in renal area and something hanged on the flank or renal area associated with haematuria. Patient also complaint of pain in testis of affected side.

According to *Nuh bin Mansoor* cause of formation of stone in kidney and bladder is constriction of neck of these organs. The *hararat* is increased, viscid and raw material is come towards these organ via urine. If excessive movement (*harkat*) is present then it converts the *rutoobat* into viscid. At beginning small particles are collected and after long period these are formed the stone.

According to *Ibn Sena* stone formation needs two things, *ghaleez madda* and stasis of these *ghaleez madda*. He said cause of formation of kidney stone and bladder stones are same, both are associated with *sabab-e-fayeli*. Two things are responsible for development of kidney, one is madda which is ready to accept the property to convert into stone and other is *quwat* which convert the *madda* into stone. The *madda* is *rutoobat* or liquid which is viscous and either from *balgham* or from *dam*. Sometimes the origin of stone formation is injury of the kidney, so the injured area can cause the collection of morbid matter at that site of the kidney.

Jalinoos said, the stone formation in kidney is due to injury while the *reem* not excrete and collect in the kidney and formed stone. Stone and microlith or *reem* formation in kidney is caused by viscid fluid of kidney and this fluid is dried and collected, formed stone. The main cause of the stone is *ghaleez madda* which is dried by the *hararat shadeed*. Thus due to *hararat* the *rutoobat* of the *madda* is dried and formed stone. In case of disturbed kidney function, the improper filtration and excretion of the urine cause the collection of urinary particles in the cavity of the kidney which may cause formation of stone.

Review of Literature

Historical Background

Renal stone disease has affected the human being from millions of years. The Babylonian Talmud refers to bladder-stone disease and includes the suggestion that patients urinate on the doorstep in order to see the stone. The evidence of urinary calculi has been found in a 7000 years old Egyptian mummy. The earliest literary quotations on detailed renal stone disease, describing symptoms and prescribing treatments to dissolve the stone, are observed within the medical texts of Asutu in Mesopotamia between 3200 and 1200 BC. The history of urinary stones almost begins and goes parallel with the history of civilization. Ancient Greeks did the first remarkable observation and documentation on urinary stone disease.

The association of stones and putrefaction has been known since Hippocrates (460–377 BC). He first described diseases of the kidney and defined symptoms of bladder stones. In his famous Oath of Medical Ethics for physicians, he underlines "I will not cut for the stone, but will leave this to be done by practitioners of this work." Hippocrates stated that wounds of the bladder were lethal. He identify both renal and bladder stone and gives the instruction for management of stones by plenty of oral fluids and diuretics.

The Assyrian Book of Medicine (300 B.C.) includes much of Hippocrates teaching. Many prescriptions are presents which mentioned the management as flushing out or dissolving renal stones. Ammonius of Alexandria (276 BC) was the first person to suggest crushing the stone to facilitate its removal. He stabilized the hook and then split the stone using a thin blunt ended instrument. Since he was the first to use the word "lithotomus" referring to cutting the stone, he was given that nickname. However, his idea did not gain popularity at that time. The first recorded details of "perineal lithotomy" were those of Cornelius Celsus (25 BC– 40 AD), who lived in Rome and wrote an encyclopedia of medicine (De Medicina). Although he, as a physician, never performed the operation himself, his description of perineal lithotomy was a landmark in the history of urology. This technique, aptly called the "Operation Minor" or "petit appareil", was used with very little change, indeed if any, for the next 1500 years. Celsus recommended the procedure to be carried out in spring, between ages of 9 and 14, with the help of two strong as well as intelligent assistants. Calus Plinus Secundus (23–79 AD), Galen (131–200 AD), and Paul of Aegine (625–690 AD) were other outstanding Greek physicians, who were practicing lithotomy, basically as described by Celsus.

Rufus gave detailed instructions for removal of bladder stones through a transverse perineal incision. With advancement of these procedure, Galen described lateral perineal lithotomy and noted the frequent occurrence of bladder stone in young boys. Rhazes in tenth century described both renal and bladder stones. He wrote book in which detail about renal stone disease with sign and symptoms. He also mentioned the medicinal and surgical treatment, the increase salt intake and hot weather are risk factors for formation of renal stone.

In the ancient times, *Iranian Muslim* physicians had performed numerous experiments concerning the urinary tract system and had acquired valuable knowledge and clinical expertise in this field. Causes of retention of urine are clearly referenced in *Rhazes' Al-Hawi* (854 to 932, AD), *Avicenna's Al-Canon* (980 to 1037, AD), and *Jurjani's Zakhira e Khwarazm shahi* (1041 to 1136, AD). In writings of *ancient Iranian physicians*, topics like oliguria, anuria, and kidney calculus disease are mentioned in detail. Analysis of urine, as the first bodily fluid to be examined, has been described in detail and provided medicine with an increasing extent of knowledge about the workings of inner bodily functions.

Albucasis (Abul Qasim Alzahrawi, 930–1013 AD) famous unani surgeon from Cordova demonstrated considerable experience in surgery by modifying the technique of lithotomy as practiced by *Ancient Greeks*. The operation was carried out through a perineal incision down to, then through, the bladder neck to reach the stone and extract it. Comparing the descriptions of the operative technique as carried out during ancient Indian and Greek civilizations, the description given by *Albucasis*. He having deep study in surgical diseases. *Al-Tasreef* famous book written by *Zehravi* clearly shows how he remarkably improved the technique of operation for removal of stone and reduced its risk. Albucasis also invented a new lithotomy scalpel, called "nechil", with 2 sharp cutting edges and being a novel instrument not known before him he made a drawing for it. The scalpel, called *"Novacula"* used by the Italian surgeon "Marianus Sanctus" in the 16th century, and the scalpel, used by the English surgeon "Shelsden" in the 18th century, were very close in shape to *Albucasis'* scalpel. Furthermore, in the ancient and Greco-Roman texts before Albucasis, there is no such emphasis on avoiding the midline perineal incision. That innovation in the technique of perineal cystolithotomy, introduced by *Albucasis*, was of considerable practical anatomical significance. Albucasis was also the first to use forceps to extract a bladder stone. Before him, extraction of the stone was by an instrument similar to a small spoon that goes around the stone and scoops it out.

In Europe, during Renaissance, most of the well-known lithotomists such as the Italian "Marianus Sanctus" (16th century AC), the French "Jack De Beaulieu" (17th century AC), and the English "Shelsden" (18th century AC) were using Albucasis' lateral approach incising on the left side. He is considered as the first to use a tool to confirm the presence of the stone before proceeding with the perineal cystolithotomy operation. He also introduced the 2-stage bladder stone operation in complicated cases. Albucasis' modifications and innovations spread to Europe in the middle Ages and remained widely adopted until the beginning of the eighteenth century, which witnessed the beginnings of the modern method the suprapubic, instead of the perineal, approach for the removal of bladder stones.

During the medieval period in Europe (1096–1438) there was little activity in the management of stone disease. In this era lithotomists were essentially commercial travelers moving from town to town looking for business and cutting all who came their way. Often uneducated and occasionally dishonest, some were great showmen. The procedure was generally performed in the public without anaesthesia and generally lasted a few minutes. However, lithotomists were held responsible for their bad results and fined accordingly.

In the 14th century, Chauliac (1300–1367), considered as the father of French surgery, wrote the Chirugia Magma, combining surgical influences of the Arabs, the Greeks, and his experiences. He wrote much about stone disease but never performed lithotomy, which was a dangerous operation at that time. Although some separation of surgery from the practice of medicine had begun to develop in early medieval times, this was accentuated in 1215 by the Fourth Lateran Council, a papal edict which forbade physicians from performing surgical procedures, as contact with blood or body fluids was viewed as contaminating to men. As a result, the practice of surgery was relegated to craft status with training by apprenticeship through guilds. Physicians followed a university-directed program of education, which involved knowledge of the classics and writings of ancient medical authors such as those by Galen, which allowed no independent thought or inquiry. Competition among physicians and surgeons, including the lowest group of surgical practitioners, the barbers, continued until Henry VIII signed a charter in 1540 uniting barbers and surgeons in London. This Guild of Barbers and Surgeons, forerunner of the Royal College of Surgeons, established a regulatory agency for training and certification of surgical practice, which set the stage for legitimizing surgery as a profession.

With Renaissance (1453–1600), there was a rapid increase in intellectual creativity in many fields. During this period, new procedures could be tried on criminals. As a result, Colot removed stones from a criminal by suprapubic approach in 1475. Thereafter, the Colot family in France held some kind of a monopoly of lithotomy over 2 centuries. They were members of the College of Surgery and had high reputation. However, the first major scientific improvement since Celsus and Albucasis was done by Farncisco de Romanis in 1520. He introduced a sound to identify the bladder neck, and the perineal incision was made onto the sound using a broad knife called "novacula." He also used retractors for exploration. His technique was popularized by his student Marius Sanctus, named as "Marian operation" or "Grand Appareil". A new technique of transurethral stone fragmentation and bladder irrigation are described by two Turkish physicians, Sabuncuo˘glu Serafettin and Ahi Ahmed Celebi, in 15th century. They also wrote about stone passage and dissolution in their text. In the 16th century the french surgeon Par´e also wrote detailed chapter on urinary stone disease and detailed procedure of lithotomy, but he never practiced it. He also wrote in detail about the stone patient in his book. The first recorded removal of a calculus by suprapubic lithotomy was also carried out during Renaissance by Pierre Franco in 1561, because of the extreme hazards of this approach Franco advised others not to follow his example.

The first kidney operation was also recorded in Renaissance around this time. In 1550 Cardan of Milan opened a lumbar abscess and discovered 18 stones. Jacques de Beaulieu (1651–1714) was the next major practitioner who practice the lithotomy and introduced the "lateral lithotomy". This method was further perfected and popularized by Ferre Jacques, who performed more than 5000 operations. The distended bladder moved upwards and therefore an extra peritoneal approach was possible this concept realize by two friends William Cheselden (1722) and John Douglas (1719). The surgical approaches for lithotomy to treat urolithiasis had very high risks of complications in the early 18th century. In the face of the very common and dangerous complications, the doctors and surgeons actively sought all possible solutions short of surgery and left lithotomy as the last alternative. In 18th-century Hermann Boerhaave (1668–1738) was one of the most important practitioner. He dedicated a chapter in his "Institutiones Medicae" to the treatment of urolithiasis. He mentioned in his book an increase in liquid intake, a hot bath in order to induce vasodilation and exercise. His opinion of lithotomy was last when other approaches fails "I think lithotomy is an act of pure faith". Since the beginning of 20th century the issue of informed consent has become the concern of medical researchers and recently became almost the main issue of medical treatment. In these informed consents, patients or parents signed that they understood the complications of lithotomy and that they would not complain and bring the case to suit in case of any complication. Famous historical figures who developed bladder stones include King Leopold I of Belgium, Peter the Great, Louis XIV, George IV, Oliver Cromwell, Benjamin Franklin, the philosopher Bacon, the scientist Newton, the physicians Harvey and Boerhaave, and the anatomist Scarpa. The very intelligent person Michelangelo make a drawing related to kidney stone disease. His drawing suggests that Michelangelo was likely familiar with the anatomy and function of the kidney as it was understood at that time most impressive in this regard is the mantle of the Creator in his painting of the Separation of Land and Water in the Sistine Ceiling, which is in the shape of a bisected right kidney.

In the beginning, studies on urinary calculi were developed before 1800 by Scheele (1742–1786) and Bergman (1734–1794), who firstly identified uric acid calculi. In the nineteenth century further studies on chemical characterization of urinary calculi was initiated by J.F. Heller, who in 1860 gave the ideas of chemical investigation of urinary calculi based on the color, hardness and chemical reactions performed directly on the dry material. These studies can be considered as the first step of development of modern Clinical Chemistry in renal stones. Prien's in 1947 first attempt to set up a classification of renal calculi for clinical purposes and the first effort to find the relationships between pathogenesis, structure and composition of calculi. After two decades of these studies there is no development in published papers. Thereafter detailed studies on the composition and micro morphology of renal stones are published that also contain scanning electron microscopy as a fundamental tool for renal stone which is first connections with urinary parameters were established. Before that there is no such type of parameters is available for kidney stones. Finally, in 1993, Daudon et al. established the first classification of renal calculi with a clear correlation with the main urinary etiologic conditions. However, this information is complex and probably is difficult to adapt to clinical routine practice, in spite of its interest for scientific purposes. Consequently, it is necessary to establish a classification of renal calculi, in accordance to its composition and fine structure, clearly correlated with specific pathophysiological conditions as the main urinary alterations, adapted to the common clinical practice. In 1874, Bigelow developed a stronger and harder lithotrite, which was introduced into the bladder with the help of anaesthesia. This procedure was called "litholapaxy." in which he filled the bladder, crushed the stone and evacuated the fragments. Due to that procedure the mortality rate decreases from 25% to 2.4%.

First planned Nephrectomy for a fistula was performed by Gustav Simon in1869. First nephrotomy carried out by Ingalls from Boston in 1873. The first pyelotomy was performed by Heinecke in 1879, and the first nephrolithotomy was carried out by Le Dentu in 1881. First to suture a nephrotomy incision was given by Czerny in 1887. First partial nephrectomy for stone disease was carried out by Kummel and Bardenheuer in 1889. In 1901 Max bordel described the avascular area of kidney which very helpful in surgery to reduce bleeding. In 1913 pyelolithotomy suggesting that it may be a safer and easier method than nephrolithotomy for removing renal stones. Extended pyelolithotomy, pioneered by Gil- Vernet in 1965 is further advancement in open renal surgery. In 1974 Fitzpatrick et al. from England further suggested the combination of extended pyelolithotomy with multiple radial nephrotomies for the treatment of large, complex staghorn stones.

The cystoscopic lithotrite develop by Young and Mckay in 1870-1945. In 1912 they were also first to perform ureteroscopy. First experience with flexible ureteroscopy using a 3mm fiberscope was given by Marshall in 1964, this was followed by Tagaki and Bush up to 1970. Rigid ureteroscopy was reported independently in 1977 by Goodman and Lyon et al. proceeding the advances in intracorporeal lithotripsy in 1980. Electrohydraulic lithotripsy was the first modern intracorporeal lithotripter invented in 1954 by Yutkin, an engineer from Kiev and popularized in 1967. Early users reported severe complications such as perforation, these were followed by successful reports of bladder stone treatment from Europe and USA (1977). Mulvaney in 1953 used the ultrasound for the destruction of urinary stones, applied by Kurth in 1977.

The development of laser for the fragmentation of ureteric calculi was initiated in 1986 and advancement in this procedure by many practitioner. Pneumatic lithotripsy is the newest technique approved for the fragmentation of renal, ureteric and bladder calculi. The first pneumatic device, the Lithoclast, was designed by a Swiss company in 1992. With improvement in renal stone surgery intracorporeal lithotripsy also allowed renal stones to be treated by percutaneous renal surgery. In 1941 Rupel and Brown removed a stone through a nephrostomy tract, Trattner in 1948 used a cystoscope to examine the renal collecting system at open renal surgery. In 1955 for purpose of draining grossly hydronephrotic kidney nephrostomy tube was placed by Goodwin et al. In 1976 Fernstrom and Johannson established percutaneous access with specific intention of removing a renal stone. Advancement in endoscopes and other instruments allowed urologists to refine the percutaneous nephrolithotomy technique during 1970s and large series were reported in 1980s.

However, with the introduction of the first ESWL machine, Dornier HM-3, in 1980, a dramatic change in stone management was observed. The US Food and Drug Administration approved the use of ESWL machines in 1984, and thereafter it was used widespread all over the world. All these improvements in the management of urinary stone disease have prevented renal damage and related renal failure due to stone to a great extent. With the subsequent developments in endourology there is an ongoing search for even less invasive treatments, and improvement in parallel with scientific development has brought us to a point where we try not to "cut" our patients for stone disease, as Hippocrates admonishes, and rather manage them with minimal invasive alternatives. Currently, open surgery is performed in less than 4% of patients with urinary stones in referral centres. Subsequent developments in urology include the introduction of percutaneous nephrolithotomy (PCNL) and the search for even less invasive treatments for stones, leading to the use of various energy sources for stone fragmentation; these milestones are listed in following table.

Table .**Developments of lithotripsy over the last century**

Method/year	Detail
PCNL 1955	Goodwin; the first percutaneous nephrostomy
1976	Dilatation of the channel to aid stone extraction
Ultrasonic lithotripsy 1953	Mulvaney discovered the sound waves that fragmented stones.
1977	Kurth first applied the technique to renal stones
Electrohydraulic lithotripsy 1913	Wappler states: 'When this spark is brought into contact with both the hard and soft species of bladder calculi, it causes them to disintegrate' Yutkin obtains a patent for electrohydraulic shock Waves.
1950 1967	URAT-1 is displayed and popularize
Laser lithotripsy 1961	Development of Nd:YAG, a solid state laser
Pneumatic or ballistic lithotripsy 1992	Swiss Lithoclast described

ESWL	
1966	Dornier employee touched a plate hit by a high velocity projectile and described an electric shock
1973	First in vitro destruction of stone reported.
1980	First patient treated with Dornier HM-1 lithotripter.
1983	First commercially available lithotripter, Dornier HM-3

Urolithiasis has its roots deeply embedded in the urological literature. Treatments have changed drastically over the centuries, from litholytic agents that dissolve calculi to open surgical procedures to remove bladder calculi. Even lithotomy has progressed from entry through the perineum, then suprapubically and finally endoscopically. Such controversy has surrounded the history of stone disease that Shakespeare commented, 'Blessed be the man who spares these stones and cursed be the man who moves these bones' (Shakespeare's own epitaph).

Surgery to the kidney was not really accepted until the 19th century, and it is only in the last few years that 95% of stones that previously required open surgery are being treated with more conservative measures. This has become possible as a result of the technological advances, scientific discoveries and questioning minds.

EPIDEMIOLOGY

PREVALENCE

Urinary calculi are one of the most common urological problems all the over world. They are particularly common in some geographical areas such as United States, South Africa, India and other South East Asian Countries. The rates of prevalence are 1 to 5% in Asia, 5 to 9% in Europe, 13% in North America, and 20% in Saudi Arabia. The stone composition and their location are not same in all countries. Recent studies using the National Health and Nutrition Examination Survey (NHANES) have suggested that the prevalence of stone disease increased from 3.8 to 5.2% Nationwide.

Disease of renal calculi is known to be one of the oldest diseases that leading to hospitalization and surgery according to need. In 1980, the percentage of population, which had the incidence of stones in USA, Sweden, Germany, Italy and UK was found to be 12.0, 9.5, 6.8, 3.1 and 1.5 respectively. In the United States the probability of formation of the renal calculi in the adult population is 2%. Southeast Asia has the paediatric problem of bladder stone found to be a continuous problem. In India it affects nearly 2 million people every year and the life time risk is about 20% in those having this disorder. Northern part of India is defined as the stone forming belt and the incidence is low in Southern part. Urolithiasis is found to be a multifactorial disorder. Decreased daily fluid intake, dry and hot climate especially in some geographical locations, are the factors which take part in formation of stone. In many countries, the geographical distribution of renal calculi is uneven. So a precise knowledge of the epidemiological factors and composition of the urinary stones with respect to the geographical location is essential for suggesting a better method of treatment and also to avoid the factors which could influence their recurrence.

Kidney stone disease varies in frequency and stone type between different climates and racial groups. Understanding the epidemiology of stones disease is important to determine the significance of the disease at a community level, the associations and risk factors for individuals and the likelihood of stone recurrence. People living in tropical belt or "stone belt", like India are those who suffer from renal stone illness resulting from rising temperatures and profuse sweating. Geographical factors combined with improper hydration, genetics, gender, diet and obesity increase the risk of formation of stones. "Stone belt" stretching from Egypt and Sudan through the Middle East, India, Pakistan, Burma, Thailand, Indonesia and Philippines reporting consistently high incidence of urolithiasis. The calculus disease in India though seen in every state is more prevalent in Gujarat, Rajasthan, Madhya Pradesh, and parts of Andhra Pradesh. Recurrence of stone disease is common with these the recurrence interval between each episode reduces. The clinical presentation of stone disease may not differ much even though different in composition.

The Occurrence of renal calculi varies with the population studied and rates of Nephrolithiasis vary regionally. Symptomatic Nephrolithiasis in 3 to 12% of the population will develop during their lifetime, more frequently in male than female, approximately 13% in men and 7% in women, especially observed in whites. Stones may present at any age, however young and middle-aged adults are more commonly affected, predominantly age 18-45 years with peak in the late 20s and early 30s, especially in hot climates and in patients of greater age. The typical presentation is mainly in the working age group (between 20 and 60 years of age). Approximately 50% of patients present between the age of 30 and 50 years. When researchers analysed data from the NHANES, they found the highest incidence of stones to be among Caucasian males (12.8 percent). Among adults ages 60 and older, 20 percent of men and 10 percent of women had a history of kidney stones. It is rare in children's, it shows a familial predisposition. In addition, its recurrence rate is also elevated. Once diagnosed, 50% of adult urolithiatic patients have recurrence in 5-10 years and 75% in 20 years.

The lifetime prevalence of kidney stone disease is estimated at 1% to 15%. The probability of having a stone varying according to age, gender, race, and geographic location. In the United States, the prevalence of stone disease has been estimated at 10% to 15%. Using data derived from the United States National Health and Nutrition Examination Survey dataset (NHANES II and III), Stamatelou and colleagues (2003) established a 5.2% prevalence of kidney stone disease from 1988 to 1994, which represents a 37% increase from 1976 to 1980 for which a 3.8% prevalence rate was determined. The finding of an increase in the prevalence of stone disease has been observed by others.

Age & Sex

Stone occurrence is relatively uncommon before the age of 20, but peaks incidence in the fourth to sixth decades of life. It has been observed that women show a bimodal distribution of stone disease, demonstrating a second peak in incidence in the sixth decade of life, corresponding to the onset of menopause. This finding, and the lower incidence of stone disease in women compared with men, has been attributed to the protective effect of estrogen against stone formation in premenopausal women, owing to enhanced renal calcium absorption and reduced bone resorption. Indeed, Heller and colleagues (2002) identified lower urinary saturation of calcium oxalate in women compared with men. Moreover, urinary calcium was lower in women than in men until age 50, after which it reached equivalence in the two groups. Estrogen-treated postmenopausal women had lower urinary calcium and saturation of calcium oxalate than untreated women.

Alternatively, Fan and associates (1999) found that androgens increased and estrogen decreased urinary and serum oxalate in an experimental rat model, perhaps accounting for the reduced risk of stone formation in women.

In Unani system of Medicine the renal calculus is named as "*Hasat-e-Kulliya*". According to Unani literature renal calculi are more common in middle-aged individuals, and bladder calculi are more common in adolescents. In middle-aged people, *harārat* (heat) is less and *khilt balgham* is more. Furthermore, the digestive power of middle-aged is weak. The lumen of the urinary tract becomes narrow due to increased *burūdat* (cold). As a result, smaller constituents pass through the kidney and into the ureter and bladder, but larger constituents retain in the kidney spaces. *Harārat* in the kidney is sufficient to dry the constituent and facilitate the formation of stones. In adolescents, the bladder calculi are usually large because they are physically more active, consume an improper diet frequently, and do not take rest after eating. In adolescence, the spaces in the kidney and urinary tract are large and open; thus urine along with its constituents easily passes from the kidney to the bladder. The *harārat-i-ghariziyā* (innate heat) is present more in adolescents and *quwwat-i dāfi'ya* (evacuating power) is also stronger in comparison with other age groups. Therefore, all the morbid matter is expelled out from the kidney along with the urine easily. In adolescence the urethral orifice and other excretory organs are small, and the constituents of the urine that are smaller in size are excreted out easily, but larger constituents remain back in the bladder. The *hararat* (heat) of the bladder acts on and dries up these constituents, thereby forming bladder stones. In case of young adults since their organs are well developed, they have more hararat compared to rutoobat in the body and all the systems i.e. digestive, excretory etc are functionally excellent. They maintain healthy dietary habits, even if morbid matter gets accumulated this is expelled out easily. In the case with females, the urethral orifice is large which facilitates easy expulsion of larger morbid matters present in urine; hence they are less prone to urolithiasis.

Isma'il Jurjani in his book *zhakhira-i-Khwarazm Shahi* states that urolithiasis is common in children, middle age and less common among elders. In children and elderly stone is formed in the bladder while in adults, in the kidneys. The causes mentioned by *Jurjānī* are that the orifices and vessels are wide in older age group whereas in case of adult they are small and tight. In case of females since they have a wider urethra compared to males, the accumulated morbid matter is easily expelled whereas in case of males the morbid matter gets accumulated and is not easily expelled. The cause for bladder stone in children is that the *quwwat-i dafi'ya* (evacuating power) is more powerful in children hence after digestion the matter is passed on to the kidney quickly and then to the bladder. Moreover, the urine of children is thick, viscid due to improper eating habits, urethral orifice is small and the salt content in the urine is more. The *ghaliz* rutoobat acted upon by the hararat causes evaporation of liquid leading to solidification of its constituents. In children the urine contains lots of sediments and the hararat is also relatively more which encourages the solidification of sediments. The main causes leading to stone formation are the excess of *ghaliz* and *lazuj* rutoobat which is formed due to *ghaliz giza*. Heavy diet such as beef, camel's meat, fried egg, Nan, wheat, milk, rice, *paneer, faluda, turanj,* guava and alcohol are the important and indirect cause of stone formation. Irregular food habits, sexual activity especially when the liver and GIT are weak and excessive hararat in the kidney are also responsible for stone formation.

According to *Hakim Azam Khan,* stones are often formed in kidneys of obese people, while in the bladder of lean people. In old age renal calculi are more common while in children and young people bladder calculi are more often found. Calculi are often formed in children because of excess and untimely eating habits, increased hararat due to growing age, their ureters are stiff and spaces are not wide open while in old age the main cause of calculi is the weakness of *quwwat-i hazima* (Digestive power).

According to *Ibn Sīnā* there are differences in the constituents of renal and bladder stones. The renal calculi are soft, small and usually reddish in color whereas the bladder stones are hard, large and sandy white or black in color. A group of *atibbā'* (Unani physicians) have mentioned that calculi formation takes place even in intestines, colon, liver and joints. Though the sediments differ in color, sometimes they are dark yellowish, sometimes red, sometimes muddy, and sometimes similar to the color of seeds of pomegranate.

The explanations given by *Sabit bin Qurra* (901 AD), *Al - Razi* (932 AD), *Ibn Sina* (1037 AD) and *Ibn Zuhar* (1162 AD) about the formation of stones were basically similar, that heavy food stuff, dairy products and poor kidney function could be the cause. They thought outflow obstruction and familial tendency are also the cause of formation of stone. All these explanations correlate with the modern concept of urolithiasis.

Race

Racial differences in the incidence of stone disease have been observed. Among U.S. men, Soucie and colleagues (1994) found the highest prevalence of stone disease in whites, followed by Hispanics, Asians, and African Americans, who had prevalence of 70%, 63%, and 44% of whites, respectively. Among U.S. women, the prevalence was highest among whites but lowest among Asian women (about half that of whites). Others found an even higher differential (threefold to fourfold) between whites and African Americans. Interestingly, despite differences in prevalence of stone disease according to ethnicity, Maloney and colleagues (2005) observed a remarkably similar incidence of metabolic abnormalities between white and non-white stone formers from the same geographic region, although the distribution of abnormalities differed, suggesting that dietary and other environmental factors may outweigh the contribution of ethnicity in determining stone risk. The gender distribution of stone disease varies according to race. Sarmina and colleagues (1987) noted a male-to-female ratio among whites of 2.3 and among African Americans of 0.65. Michaels and coworkers (1994) also noted a reversal of the male predisposition to stone disease in Hispanics and African Americans, reporting a male-to-female ratio of 1.8 among Asians, 1.6 among whites, 0.7 among Hispanics, and 0.5 among African Americans, among a group of patients undergoing extracorporeal shock wave lithotripsy. Soucie and associates (1994) observed a similar trend in the male-to-female ratio of the lifetime incidence of stone disease of 3.4 among Asians, 2.6 among whites, 2.1 among Hispanics, and 1.8 among African Americans, although the actual ratios differed in the two studies. Dall'era and colleagues (2005) reviewed emergency department records to identify patients presenting with symptomatic renal or ureteral calculi and found a male to female ratio of 1.17 among Hispanic patients compared with 2.05 for white patients.

Geography

The geographic distribution of stone disease tends to roughly follow environmental risk factors, a higher prevalence of stone disease is found in hot, arid, or dry climates such as the mountains, desert, or tropical areas. However, genetic factors and dietary influences may outweigh the effects of geography. Finlayson (1974) reviewed several worldwide geographic surveys and found that areas of high stone prevalence included the United States, British Isles, Scandinavian and Mediterranean countries, northern India and Pakistan, northern Australia, Central Europe, portions of the Malay Peninsula, and China. Within the United States, Mandel and Mandel (1989a, 1989b) identified the highest rates of hospital discharge for patients with calcium oxalate stones in the Southeast and for uric acid stones in the East, among the veteran patient population. Soucie and associates (1994) found increasing age-adjusted prevalence rates in both men and women going from north to south and west to east, with the highest prevalence observed in the Southeast. After controlling for other risk factors, the authors determined that ambient temperature and sunlight were independently associated with stone prevalence.

Climate

Seasonal variation in stone disease is likely related to temperature by way of fluid losses through perspiration and perhaps by sunlight-induced increases in vitamin D. Prince and Scardino (1960) noted the highest incidence of stone disease in the summer months, July through September, with the peak occurring within 1 to 2 months of maximal mean temperatures (Prince et al, 1956). Likewise, Bateson (1973) reported a peak incidence of stone disease between December and March in Australia, corresponding to the summer season. The study of military personnel translocated to desert locations has provided a unique opportunity to study the effect of climate on a defined population. Pierce and Bloom (1945) reported that American soldiers in an undisclosed desert location had an increase in symptomatic episodes of renal colic during the summer season. Another study of military personnel who developed symptomatic stones after arrival in Kuwait and Iraq disclosed a mean time interval to stone formation of 93 days. Finally, Parry and Lister (1975) measured urinary calcium and magnesium levels in soldiers before and 10 days after transfer to the Persian Gulf and noted increased urinary calcium levels from baseline in those soldiers transferred during the summer months but not among those transferred during the "cold season," which was attributed to sunlight-induced increased production of 1,25-dihydroxy cholecalciferol (1,25[OH]2D3). Thus it is likely that climate and geography influence the prevalence of stone disease indirectly, through effects on temperature and possibly sunlight.

Occupation

Heat exposure and dehydration constitute occupational risk factors for stone disease as well. Cooks and engineering room personnel, both of whom are exposed to high temperatures, were found to have the highest rates of stone formation among personnel of the Royal Navy. Likewise, Atan and colleagues (2005) found a significantly higher incidence of stones among steel workers exposed to high temperatures (8%) compared with those working in normal temperatures (0.9%). Metabolic evaluation of these two groups of workers showed a higher incidence of low urine volume and hypocitraturia among the workers in the hot area. Borghi and colleagues (1993) also noted differences in the incidence of stone disease and urinary stone risk factors among workers at a glass plant who were or were not chronically exposed to high temperatures causing massive perspiration. Those exposed to high temperatures exhibited lower urine volumes and pH, higher uric acid levels, and higher urine specific gravity, leading to higher urinary saturation of uric acid. Accordingly, those workers who formed stones had a remarkably high incidence of uric acid stones (38%).

Individuals with sedentary occupations, such as those in managerial or professional positions, have been found to carry an increased risk of stone formation for unclear reasons. This finding is consistent with the work of Robertson and associates, who reported an increased risk of stone disease in affluent individuals, countries, and societies, which may be reflective of a more indulgent diet and lifestyle.

Body Mass Index and Weight

The association of body size and incidence of stone disease has been investigated. In two large prospective cohort studies of men and women, the prevalence and incident risk of stone disease were directly correlated with weight and body mass index in both sexes, although the magnitude of the association was greater in women than men. Although these investigators identified a reduced risk of incident stone formation with high intake of fluid (men and women) and low protein intake (men), they found that obesity and weight gain were independent risk factors for incident stone formation and could not be accounted for by diet alone. Recent evidence linking obesity and insulin resistance with low urine pH and uric acid stones as well as an association between hyperinsulinemia and hypercalciuria could account for an increased risk of uric acid and/or calcium stones in obese patients.

Water

The beneficial effect of a high fluid intake on stone prevention has long been recognized. In two large observational studies, fluid intake was found to be inversely related to the risk of incident kidney stone formation. Furthermore, in a prospective, randomized trial assessing the effect of fluid intake on stone recurrence among first-time idiopathic calcium stone formers, urine volume was significantly higher in the group assigned to a high fluid intake compared with the control group receiving no recommendations, and, accordingly, stone recurrence rates were significantly lower (12% vs. 27%, respectively). Geographic differences in the incidence of stone disease have been ascribed in some cases to differences in the mineral and electrolyte content of water in different areas. Although several investigators reported a lower incidence of stone disease in geographic regions with a "hard" water supply compared with a "soft" water supply, where water "hardness" is determined by content of calcium carbonate, others found no difference. Schwartz and coworkers (2002) found no association between water hardness and incidence of stone episodes, although they did observe a correlation between water hardness and urinary magnesium, calcium, and citrate levels.

More water intake less chances of stone formation.

DEFINITION

UROLITHIASIS = stone in renal system (stone like body formation)

NEPHROLITHIASIS = stone in kidney

URETEROLITHIASIS = stone in ureter

CYSTOLITHIASIS = stone in urinary bladder

Nephrolithiasis—from the *Greek* word nephros, meaning "kidney" and *lithos*, meaning "stone"—refers to the condition of having stones in the kidney or collecting system.

Kidney stones can form when substances in the urine—such as calcium, oxalate, and phosphorus—become highly concentrated. Nephrolithiasis or kidney stone disease, is a condition in which individuals form calculi (stones) within the renal pelvis and tubular lumens Renal stone is a crystalline mass or a concretions or a solid accumulations of material that formed by precipitation of various urinary solutes in the tubal system of the kidney. It can vary in size from as small as grains of sand to large as golf ball.

Urolithiasis, or urinary calculus are crystalline aggregates of one or more components of the urine, most commonly calcium oxalate. They also may contain calcium phosphate, magnesium ammonium phosphate (struvite), uric acid, or cystine. Calcium and struvite containing stones often are visible on plain radiographs, but CT scans will demonstrate all calculi. Nephrocalcinosis and uro-(nephro-) lithiasis frequently coexist and the terms are often loosely combined when describing patients with urinary stone disease. Whether they are aetiologically distinct is unclear, although it is generally believed that nephrocalcinosis represents one end of the spectrum of urinary stone disease. However, although nephrocalcinosis is often associated with urinary stones, most patients with urinary stones do not have macroscopic nephrocalcinosis. Urolithiasis is one of the most common disease of urinary tract. Urinary calculus is stone like body composed of urinary salts bound together by a colloid matrix of organic materials. It consist of a nucleus around which concentric layers of urinary salts are deposited. Nephrolithiasis is defined as the occurrence of stones in the collecting system of the kidney. Nephrolithiasis is a condition in which organic and inorganic masses form within the urinary tract. Stone formation may occur when the urinary concentration of crystals (e.g. calcium, oxalate and uric acid) is high and when the concentration of substances that inhibit stone formation (e.g. citrate) is low. The development of urinary calculi or kidney stones is known as urolithiasis or nephrolithiasis.

ETIOLOGY

Renal stone disease occurs worldwide and has been recognised as a medical problem even from the BC era. Urine contains various solute dissolved in water. The concentration of urine changes depending on the amount of water and solutes. When the concentration of solutes in urine increases, it reaches a state of saturation. (Saturation is the point at which the water and the minerals dissolved in the urine are in equilibrium and precipitation does not occur below this level and further increase in solute load leads to supersaturation). Supersaturation is the level beyond which addition of further solute invariably result in crystallisation. Idiopathic renal urolithiasis accounts for 60-80% of stone disease. Stone formation occurs when normally soluble material (e.g., calcium) supersaturates the urine and begins the process of crystal formation. In the formation of renal stone multiple factors are involved.

Approximately 80% of kidney stones contain calcium, and the majority of them are composed primarily of calcium oxalate. Although most calcium oxalate stones contain some calcium phosphate, only5% have hydroxyapatite or brushite as their main constituent and 10% contain some uric acid. Pure uric acid, cystine and infection stones are less common. Although composition of each stone correlates with supersaturation values in the urine (16), calculi are seldom found without an admixture of many salts and not every passed stone can be retrieved for chemical analysis. In addition, patients may present multiple stones and in case of persistence of small and non-obstructive calculi after spontaneous elimination or surgical removal, the calculi might not present exactly the same admixture as the voided or removed ones. Since the prevention is aimed to avert new stone formation and further growth of the remaining calculi, evaluation of patients should be rather directed toward identifying urinary risk factors for stone formation or recurrence with the goal of devising appropriate, individualized therapy. Evaluation of a renal stone patient starts with a detailed history focusing on occupation, dietary and lifestyle habits, previous use of medications, family predisposition, and history of recurrent urinary tract infection and underlying disorders that predisposes to nephrolithiasis. Incidental finding of asymptomatic stones on a radiograph/ultra-sound may also occur. The majority of calcium oxalate stone formers (SF) suffers from no systemic disease and can be described as idiopathic calcium oxalate SF patients. Metabolic abnormalities responsible for stone recurrence are currently identified in up to 90% of such patients and will be the focus of the present review.

The cause of renal stone formation is not yet fully understood but in majority of cases multiple factors are involved. The important factors which influence the formation and growth of uroliths are as follows:—

METABOLIC EVALUATION

A complete or comprehensive urinary metabolic profile to guide prophylaxis of stone recurrence, consisting of two 24-hr urine samples for stone risk analysis as well as an oral calcium load test has been advocated lately to be time-consuming and expensive.

In a very recent cost-effectiveness analysis of medical management strategies for nephrolithiasis by the group of Park and his associates, such comprehensive or detailed metabolic evaluation offered no advantage in cost or efficacy over a simple metabolic evaluation (single 24-hr urine collection) with respect to treatment of recurrent stone formers. Therefore, a simple metabolic evaluation consisting of a single 24-hour urine collection for analysis of all urinary stone risk factors may be sufficient for a medical evaluation of urolithiasis. On the other hand, Parks et al, and others reported that only one 24-hour urine specimen may lead to misdiagnosis of common metabolic disturbances.

The routine laboratorial investigation among urolithiasis patients includes the determination of urinary parameters involved in stone formation such as urinary calcium, oxalate, magnesium, citrate, uric acid, sodium, potassium and creatinine. Spot urine for urinary sediment and culture to rule out urinary tract infection are also part of the investigation. Urinary pH must be determined in a 12-hr fasting sample and a venous blood gas analysis must be obtained to screen for complete forms of distal Renal Tubular Acidosis. When systemic acidosis is not present, an ammonium chloride test is needed. A blood sample must be obtained for serum creatinine, calcium (total or ionized), phosphate and uric acid determinations. Bone mineral density has to be assessed mainly among idiopathic hypercalciuria patients, due to the important association of urinary calcium losses with low bone mineral density. Since primary hyperparathyroidism has to be ruled out, serum PTH can be determined either in the same single blood collection or in a further sample in case hypercalcemia has been detected in the former, in order to reduce costs. However, intermittent high levels of serum calcium may represent mild forms of subtle primary hyperparathyroidism. A qualitative colorimetric test in spot urine samples to evidence the presence of high amounts of cystine with sodium nitroprussiate can serve as a screening method for cystinuria

HYPEREXCRETION OF RELATIVELY INSOLUBLE URINARY CONSTITUENTS

Oxalate

Though oxalate is the major component of 70% of all renal stones, yet hyperoxaluria as a cause of formation of such stone is relatively rare Cabbage, rhubarb, spinach, tomatoes, black tea and cocoa contain large amount of oxalate. Ingestion of excessive amounts of ascorbic acid and orange juice also increase urinary oxalate excretion. But dietary oxalate is usually poorly absorbed and does not play a major role in formation of oxalate stones. In fact restriction of these foods has limited effect in prevention of oxalate stones. Primary hyperoxaluria is a rare genetic disorder affecting the metabolism of glyoxylic acid, which forms oxalate rather than other soluble end products. It is an important cause of nephrolithiasis in children. Acquired forms of hyperoxaluria include pyridoxine deficiency, ethylene glycol poisoning small bowel disease with hyperabsorption of dietary oxalate and methoxyflurane anaesthesia.

Hyperoxaluria can be due to an enzymatic disturbance in oxalate biosynthesis but primary hyperoxaluria type I, the prevailing type, is a rare genetic disorder. Most cases of increased urinary oxalate found in CSF patients are represented by secondary or mild hyperoxaluria, defined by levels of urinary oxalate higher than 45 mg/day, with a reported frequency of around 12%. Secondary hyperoxaluria is due to either increased availability of substrate (ascorbic acid, ethylene glycol, methoxyflurane), reduced degradation of oxalate by intestinal bacteria or intestinal hyperabsorption of oxalate (imbalance between intraluminal calcium and oxalate as in enteric hyperoxaluria or due to a low-calcium diet). Enteric hyperoxaluria induced by fat and bile salt malabsorption is the hallmark of hyperoxaluria due to intestinal hyperabsorption of oxalate. The gastrointestinal diseases that have been associated with this entity are those characterized by an absence or nonfunctioning of the small bowel (enteritis, small bowel resection or bypass surgery) and those causing defective absorption of fat or bile acids (chronic pancreatitis, biliary cirrhosis, blind loop syndrome and other diseases). Unabsorbed bile acids and fatty acids form complexes with calcium in the intestinal lumen, limiting the amount of free calcium to bind oxalate, with a consequent increase in intestinal oxalate absorption leading to hyperoxaluria. Dietary calcium restriction may lead to hyperoxaluria through the same mechanism. Other pathophysiological conditions occurring alone in less than 2% of SF patients include distal Renal Tubular Acidosis, Infection Stones and Cystinuria.

Calcium

On regular diets normal urinary excretion of calcium ranges between 200 mg to 300 mg per day. The major calcium in foods are in milk and cheese. Milk and dietary protein also cause increased absorption of calcium from the gut. In a few conditions e.g. prolonged immobilisation and certain bone diseases (e.g. myeloma, Paget's disease and metastatic cancer) there is hypercalciuria. In these cases calcium excretion may increase upto 450 mg or more per day. Primary hyperparathyroidism also causes hypercalciuria. 2/3rd of these patients may produce renal stones. There is a condition which is called 'idiopathic hypercalciuria' in which males excrete more calcium though the serum calcium is normal and serum phosphorus is decreased. This may be due to defective renal tubular reabsorption of calcium.

Hypervitaminosis D may also cause hypercalciuria. Renal tubular acidosis also causes hypercalciuria. But in spite of this long list majority of the above conditions do not produce renal stones.

Idiopathic hypercalciuria

It is generally agreed that the oversaturation of urine with calcium is one of the most important risk factors for calcium nephrolithiasis. Primary hyperparathyroidism, the most common primary cause of resorptive hypercalciuria, hence hypercalcemia is present in less than 1% of nephrolithiasis patients. Conversely, idiopathic hypercalciuria represents the primary metabolic alteration in almost 50% of patients. Idiopathic hypercalciuria (IH) is defined by levels of urinary calcium excretion in a 24-hour urine sample exceeding 300 mg/day (7.5 mmoL) in men or 250 mg/day (6.25 mmoL) in women or higher than 4 mg (0.1 mmoL) per kilogram of body weight per day, regardless of gender and age, in the absence of hypercalcemia. However, levels around 200 mg/day or higher than 150 mg per gram of urinary creatinine can also increase supersaturation in patients with recurrent stones. The increased daily urinary excretion rate of calcium among patients with kidney stones was first recognized by Flocks in 1939 and subsequently in 1953, Albright et al. introduced the term Idiopathic Hypercalciuria (IH) to distinguish a group of calcium stone formers (CSF) who exhibited hypercalciuria without hypercalcemia, and did not have a history of excessive vitamin D use, primary hyperparathyroidism, hyperthyroidism, renal tubular acidosis, sarcosidosis, other granulomas or malignancy.

An acute oral calcium load test, described in 1975 by Pak et al, should clearly distinguish between absorptive and renal (renal calcium leak) subtypes of hypercalciuria. In a previous evaluation by our group, a 24-hr urinary calcium excretion, under conditions of a mean usual calcium intake of around 500 mg/day, was determined in CSF patients who previously presented an absorptive or renal response to this test. We observed that the majority of them, 63 and 78% of each group, presented normocalciuria rather than hypercalciuria. Since this apparently normal calcium excretion might have resulted from a combination of high calcium absorption and low calcium intake, those patients where then challenged to a higher calcium intake of 1,500 mg/day given as supplement for one week. Regardless of whether there was a former absorptive or renal-like response to the acute load, the higher calcium intake disclosed the presence of subpopulations sensitive to calcium intake in previously normocalciuric patients. Conversely, most of the hypercalciuric patients, when challenged to a higher calcium intake did not present a further increase in their urinary calcium, showing that under conditions of low calcium intake, as is the case of the Brazilian population, patients were already excreting calcium in excess of their intake, hence being considered as dietary calcium-independent. In addition, as the morning urinary fasting calcium/creatinine (Ca/Cr) ratio seemed to be the single parameter which would distinguish between renal and absorptive hypercalciuric patients, with a cut off value of 0.11, we repeated this determination in 31 patients (34) and found that 87% of them changed their results from values higher than 0.11 to lower values. Taken together, these data suggest that Absorptive and Renal Hypercalciuria should be considered the same rather than two distinct entities, a hypothesis already raised by Coe et al. representing a systemic abnormality of calcium homeostasis probably induced by a dysregulation of 1,25(OH)2D3, leading to alterations in calcium transport in the intestine, kidney and bone characterized by increased intestinal calcium absorption and bone resorption, as well as decreased renal tubular calcium reabsorption. Several series in the literature, including the one from our group have demonstrated that BMD is reduced in IH patients. Some of them have reported increase of bone resorption markers as well. A histomorphometric study undertaken by our group in 1994 disclosed a low bone volume, a tendency of low bone formation coupled with increased bone resorption and delayed bone mineralization in male hypercalciuric CSF patients. Other bone biopsy reports showed conflicting data regarding bone resorption, but all of them have suggested low bone formation and a severe mineralization defect in hypercalciuric patients (47-50). The underlying mechanisms responsible for higher bone resorption and/or lower bone formation in this setting are still unclear and the reasons for the mineralization defect remain unknown if one considers that serum levels of calcium, phosphorus and vitamin D are normal in these patients.

Anyway, a population-based study has shown a fourfold increase in vertebral fracture risk among urolithiasis patients when compared to the general population, and in a large cross sectional survey (Third National Health and Nutrition Examination Survey, NHANES III), a history of kidney stone was found to be associated with lower femoral neck BMD and more prevalent wrist and spine fractures in men after adjustments for age and body mass index. Whether idiopathic hypercalciuria is the result of a primary bone disorder, a consequence of a persisting negative calcium balance or a combination of both still remains to be determined. Nevertheless, bone status must be evaluated and followed up in patients with IH.

Uric acid: many patients with gout form uric acid calculi particularly when under treatment. If the urine is made alkaline and diluted while treating this disease chance of uric acid stone formation is less. Administration of allopurinol also decreases stone formation. Many uric acid stone formers have normal serum and urinary uric acid levels but show a consistently low urinary pH.

Hyperuricosuria and uric acid: Nephrolithiasis Hyperuricosuria is defined by uric acid excretion above 750 and 800 mg/day for women and men, respectively. Its prevalence is highly variable among different series. Hyperuricosuria may be secondary to uricosuric medications, myeloproliferative disorders, primary gout or congenital disorders. A high animal protein (especially purines) may increase uric acid excretion and decrease urinary pH. Uric acid supersaturation is strongly controlled by urinary pH. Diarrheas states may predispose to uric acid nephrolithiasis due to low urine volume and urinary pH. Uric acid may provide heterogeneous nuclei for calcium oxalate stone formation. The lower frequency of pure uric acid stones, around 5%, may be ascribed to the usual urine acidity, which favors calcium oxalate crystallization instead. However, recent findings provided by metabolic studies have indicated an association between pure uric acid nephrolithiasis and insulin resistance (53,54). Those patients present abdominal obesity, dyslipidemia, arterial hypertension, elevated fasting glucose levels and lower glucose disposal rate, hyperuricemia, normouricosuria, and low urinary pH (53). The latter may explain stone formation despite of normouricosuria. Potential mechanisms include impaired ammoniagenesis caused by resistance to insulin action in proximal tubule or substrate competition by free fatty acids.

Cystine

Cystinuria is a hereditary disease which is more common in infants and children. Only a small percentage of patients with cystinuria form stones.

Cystinuria is a rare autosomic recessive disorder characterized by reduced renal tubular reabsorption of the dibasic aminoacids cystine, ornithine, lysine and arginine (58). Overexcretion of cystine leads to stone formation because its solubility in the urine is very low under normal urine pH.

Hypocitraturia

Low urinary citrate levels below 320 mg/day, hypocitraturia, occur in approximately 50% of adult SF patients (17), isolated or associated with other metabolic disturbances. Hypocitraturia may result from distal renal tubular acidosis, chronic diarrheal syndrome, hypokalemia, urinary tract infection, but mostly it is of unknown etiology, namely idiopathic hypocitraturia. Citrate binds calcium in a soluble salt inhibiting crystallization and slowing stone formation.

Distal Renal Tubular Acidosis (dRTA)

dRTA is characterized by alkaline fasting urine pH associated to hypercloremic hypokalemic metabolic acidosis, hypocitraturia, hypercalciuria and often bone disease (24). Acquired forms may be secondary to different tubulo-interstitial renal diseases, calcium disorders, drugs and toxins, autoimmune diseases (especially Sjögren syndrome), among others. Hereditary forms are mostly associated with nephrocalcinosis.

Drug induced stone

In rare cases, the long term use of magnesium trisilicate in the treatment of peptic ulcer has produced radio-opaque silicon stones.

PHYSICAL CHANGES IN THE URINE

1. Urinary pH — the mean urinary pH is 5.85. It is influenced by diet and medicines. If the urine becomes infected with urea splitting bacteria e.g. proteus mirabilis, it makes the urine strongly alkaline by liberating ammonia. The inorganic salts which are less soluble in alkaline medium e.g. calcium phosphate and magnesium ammonium phosphate (triple phosphate) will form urinary stones.

2. Colloid content — As mentioned above it has long been claimed that the colloids in the urine allow the crystalloids to be held in a supersaturated state. But the importance of this theory has been questioned recently.

3. Decreased concentration of crystalloids— this may be due to low fluid intake, excessive water losses in febrile disease and in hot climates, due to excessive perspiration or due to excessive water loss from vomiting and diarrhoea.

4. Urinary magnesium/calcium ratio— this probably has notable influence on stone formation. Acetazolamide (Diamox) causes hypercalciuria and a decrease in the ratio — this is related to increased incidence of stone formation. The thiazides, which have tremendous influence in preventing recurrence of stone formation, increase this ratio.

C. ALTERED URINARY CRYSTALLOIDS AND COLLOIDS — in urine there are quite a number of crystalloids of different types. These crystalloids are kept in solution by the presence of colloids in the urine by the process of absorption. Urinary crystalloids are discussed below e.g. oxalate, calcium cystine, uricacidetc. Urinary colloids are mucin and chondroitin sulphuric acid,

(a) When there is imbalance in the crystalloid-colloid ratio — either there is an increase in the crystalloid level or a fall in the colloid level, urinary stones may be formed,

(b) If there is any modification of the colloids e.g. they lose their solvent action or adhesive property, urinary stones may develop.

D. DECREASED URINARY OUTPUT OF CITRATE— Presence of citrate in the urine keeps relatively insoluble calcium phosphate and carbonate in solution. The normal citrate concentration in urine is 300–900 mg 24 h (1.6–4.7 mmol 24 h) as citric acid per day. Excretion of citrate depends on certain hormones. It is decreased during menstruation.

E. VITAMIN A DEFICIENCY

Deficiency of Vitamin A in the food tends to induce stone formation in animals. Stone formation is more common in northern parts of India and Egypt probably due to this. Deficiency of Vitamin A causes desquamation of the epithelium. The desquamated cells form nidus for stone formation. This is more applicable to bladder stones.

F. URINARY INFECTION

Association of stone with infection is very intimate. In about 80% of cases there is infection of the urinary tract. But it is difficult to say whether it is the cause or result of such infection,

(a) Infection disturbs the colloid content of the urine, so there is more chance of stone formation,

(b) Infection also causes abnormality in the colloids which may cause the crystalloid to be precipitated,

(c) Infection also changes urinary pH which helps in stone formation,

(d) Infection also causes increase in concentration of crystalloids, which may under some circumstances produce stone. Infection favours the formation of urinary calculi. Clinical and experimental stone formation are common when urine is infected with urea-splitting streptococci, staphylococci and especially Proteus spp. The predominant bacteria found in the nuclei of urinary stones are staphylococci and Escherichia coli.

Infection stones form in the setting of upper urinary tract infection with urease-producing bacteria. Those microorganisms hydrolyze urea producing ammonia and hydroxide, increasing urinary pH and phosphate that bind to magnesium to form a "triple-crystal" composed of struvite (magnesium ammonium phosphate) and/or calcium carbonate apatite. Those calculi usually grow as branched stones that occupy a large portion of the collecting system, namely, staghorn calculi.

Prolonged immobilisation

Immobilisation from any cause, e.g. paraplegia, is liable to result in skeletal decalcification and an increase in urinary calcium favouring the formation of calcium phosphate calculi.

G. URINARY STASIS

It goes without saying that stones are more prone to occur when there is obstruction to the free passage of urine,

(a) Urinary stasis provides a fertile field for bacterial growth,

(b) It also causes a shift of the pH of the urine to the alkaline side,

(c) Stasis also predisposes urinary infection,

(d) It allows the crystalloids to precipitate.

H. HYPERPARATHYROIDISM

Though this condition is seen in only 2% to 5% of cases of renal stone, yet its potentiality to form urinary calculus cannot be underestimated. In cases of multiple or recurrent urinary calculi this cause should be eliminated. Due to overproduction of parathormone the bones become decalcified and calcium concentration in the urine is increased. This extra calcium may be deposited in the renal tubules or in the pelvis to form renal calculus. Peculiarly enough renal calculi are more likely to develop when hyperparathyroidism is mild and prolonged without much skeletal lesion.

A parathyroid adenoma should be removed before definitive treatment for the urinary calculi.

NIDUS OR NUCLEUS OF STONE FORMATION (Including Randall's plaque)

Randall observed that the initial lesion in formation of renal calculus is erosion at the apex of one of the renal papillae. Calcific plaques are seen on these renal papillae, which were known as Randall's plaques. He believed that this erosion developed as a result of injury secondary to infection Randall postulated that when the overlying mucosa is ulcerated, the calcification acts as a nidus on to which insoluble crystals deposit to form stones. Many investigators subsequently believed that most stones develop by precipitation of crystals e.g. calcium oxalate on an organic matrix formed of amino acids and carbohydrates. Even blood clots, clumps of epithelial cells, bacteria or even pus cells may form nidus. Necrotic ischaemic tissue and foreign bodies may form nidus and encourage stone formation. Such tissues may be caused by neoplasms, necrotic papillae or ulcerated mucous membrane from infection.

The causes of stone formation can be divided into anatomical, genetic, pathological and drug related. Large observational studies have shown that low fluid intake, low calcium intake and high fructose intake increase the risk of stone formation. Stones usually form when conditions favour separation of crystals out of the urine; many patients may have low urine volume and one or more biochemical abnormalities in the urine or blood. The most common abnormality is hypercalciuria; other abnormalities include hypercalcemia, hyperuricaemia, hyperuricosuria, hyperoxaluria, hypocitraturia, and either low or high urine pH.

Anatomical abnormalities

That occur along the urinary tract are key factors in preventing adequate flow of urine. This disturbance in flow favours the deposition of crystals and promotes stone formation. Wherever there is a change in the normal anatomical structure of the urinary tract, stone formation should be suspected, as in horseshoe kidney, medullary sponge kidneys and a calyceal diverticulum. The flow of urine from the kidney would be hindered in pelviuretric junction obstruction, ureteric stricture and ureterocele.

Genetic factors

Are considered to be the cause for half the risk of developing kidney stones. The main genetic causes are cystinuria, primary hyperoxaluria, renal tubular acidosis and Xanthinuria.

Medical conditions

That may cause stone formation include hyperparathyroidism, nephrocalcinosis and malabsorptive conditions such as Crohn's disease, intestinal resection and jejuno-ileal bypass. Patients who have had bariatric surgery are also prone to develop kidney stones. Patients with urinary diversion may develop enteric hyperoxaluria and form oxalate stones.

Dietetic Deficiency of vitamin A

Causes desquamation of epithelium. The cells form a nidus on which a stone is deposited. It is uncertain whether this mechanism is of importance other than in the formation of bladder calculi.

Basically the renal stones can be primary secondary or stones. Primary stones appear in apparently healthy urinary tract without inflammation. Usually formed in the acidic urine. These stones usually consist of calcium oxalate, uric acid, urates, cystine, xanthine, indigo, or calcium carbonate. Secondary stones are formed as the result of inflammation in the urinary tract, urine is usually alkaline. These stones are phosphate calculi and mixed stones.

Etiologic classification of Urolithiasis

1. **Hypercalcemic states**

    i. Primary hyperparathyroidism

    ii. Immobilizations

    iii. Hypervitaminosis D

    iv. Neoplasia

    v. Milk alkali syndrome

    vi. Sarcoidosis

2. **Uric acid lithiasis**

    i. Idiopathic uric acid stones

    ii. Gout

    iii. Myeloproliferative disorders

    iv. Acidic urine and oliguric state

3. **Idiopathic renal lithiasis**

    i.   With hypercalciuria

    ii.   Without hypercalciuria

    iii.   Hyperuricosuria

    iv.   Hyperoxaluria

    v.   Hypocitraturia

vi.   Increased urine alkalinity

4. Renal tubular syndrome and enzyme abnormalities

i. Distal renal tubular acidosis

ii. Carbonic anhydrase inhibitors

iii. Hyperoxaluria

iv. Cystinuria

v. Xanthinuria

5. Drugs

i. Triameterene

ii. Acyclovir

iii. Indinavir

iv. Sulphonamides

Secondary Nephrolithiasis

1. Cystic renal diseases

2. Urinary diversion procedures

3. Stents and suture materials

4. Catheters.

MECHANISM OF FORMATION OF RENAL STONES

There are numerous pathogenic theories such as the precipitation and crystallization theory (the oversaturation theory), the nucleation theory, the suppression of mechanisms of crystallization inhibition and the association of multiple mechanisms.

Studies on chemical composition of the stones indicates the following incidence:

- Calcium oxalate - the main component (75-80%)

- Calcium phosphate - 5%

- Uric acid -5%

- Struvite – magnesium ammonium phosphate and calcium phosphate - as a result of infections ≤5%

- Cystine - 1%.4

THEORIES OF STONE FORMATION

SUPERSATURATION

Urine contains various solute dissolved in water, the concentration of urine changes depending on the amount of water and solutes. When the concentration of solutes in urine increases, it reaches a state of saturation. It is the point at which the water and the minerals dissolved in the urine are in equilibrium and precipitation does not occur below this level. Further increase in solute load leads to supersaturation. The level beyond which addition of further solute invariably result in crystallisation called Supersaturation.

Nephrolithiasis is defined as the occurrence of stones in the collecting system of the kidney. It starts by the aggregation of crystals on a nidus. The nidus can be glycoprotein matrix, injured epithelium, foreign body or another crystals. Once such a nidus is formed and urine supersaturated, aggregation of crystals occur over the nidus and the crystals grows in size to form a stone.

Randall's Plaque and Microlith Theory

Randall suggested that the initial lesion in some cases of kidney stone is an erosion at the tip of a renal papilla. Deposition of calcium on this erosion produced a lesion that has been called Randall's plaque. It has further been shown that minute concretion (microliths) regularly occur in the renal parenchyma and Carr postulated that these particles are carried by lymphatic to the sub endothelial region, where they may accumulate. Ulceration of the epithelium exposes the surface, which results in precipitation and thus stone formation. The importance of Randall's plaque and Carr's microliths in most patients with stones is a matter for debate. Stone formation occurs when normally soluble material (e.g., calcium) supersaturates the urine and begins process of crystal formation. It is not clear how crystals formed in the tubules become a stone rather than being washed away by the high rate of urine flow. It is presumed that crystal aggregates become large enough to be anchored (usually at the end of the collecting ducts) and then slowly increase in size over time. This anchoring is thought to occur at sites of epithelial cell injury, perhaps induced by the crystals themselves.

PATHOPHYSIOLOGY

There are two basic aspects in the pathogenesis of renal stones:-

a) Increased urinary excretion of stone forming elements like calcium, phosphorus, uric acid, oxalate, and cystine.

b) Physiochemical changes which influence stone formation like pH of urine, stone matrix, and protective substances in the urine. For a stone to form within the urinary tract, urine must be supersaturated for precipitating crystalline component. Thus, a major consideration is the state of saturation within the urine. Solute load is important, but since urine is a complex solution, other factors influence saturation. Normally urine has presence of inorganic and organic substances which inhibit crystallisation of elements which lead to stone formation. These agents can modify nucleation, crystallisation, and aggregation. PH of the urine can also influence stone formation. When calcium and oxalate is mixed in water at stable temperature it remains in dissolved state, addition of further calcium or oxalate which increases its concentration would lead to the growth of preformed crystals but the solution remains clear. This phase is called metastable state. Further addition of calcium and or oxalate will lead to appearance of solid form or stone. This state of solution is called supersaturation.

In Unani system of Medicine the renal calculus is named as *"Hasat-e-Kulliya"*. Ancient literatures described broadly the pathology, manifestations and treatment of *Hasat-e-kulliya*. According to *Ali Ibn Abbas al-Majusi* Renal calculi are due to *shadid Hararat/* increase *hararat ghareeziya* of the kidney and *ghaliz khilt* in the body. The *shadid hararat* evaporate the moisture within the *ghaliz khilt* and the dried constituents form stones over a period of time. The formation of renal calculi depends on the viscosity of the *khilt ghaliz* following interaction with *shadid hararat*. A moderate increase in viscosity results in the formation of Reeg (crest), which is not as hard as renal calculi and is slowly excreted from the urinary tract along with urine and forms sediments in the urine. However, a significant increase in viscosity results in the formation of very hard and large particles, which are not as readily excreted and combine to form renal calculi. The persistence of *shadid hararat* in the kidneys leads to hardening of the stones, when stones retain in the urinary tract for a long period of time with these if there is constriction in pathway of urine or ureter (*majari*) cause the accumulation of small crystals and further it forms stone.

Ibn al-'Abbas al-Majusi also notes that the formation of *hasat masana* (bladder calculi) is similar to that of renal calculi. Bladder calculi are commonly seen in adolescents because they are more prone to *ratab mizāj*, are more physically active, and consume an improper diet, whereas in adults bladder calculi are common in those who consume heavy diet.

According to *Jalinoos* renal stones are formed when *riyah* is trapped in the spaces of the kidney and consolidates into hard substances. Another cause of renal calculi is ulceration of the kidney, in which pus accumulates and solidifies, thereby forming renal stones or at least establishing a nidus for the formation of stones.

Avicenna contends that the persistence of "morbid matter" in the urinary tract is instrumental in the formation of *ghalīz māddā*. Morbid matter is formed when a heavy diet is consumed; foods in such diet include thick milk, paneer (cheese), fried meat, rice, flour and fruits that are not easily digested. These foods produce a thick, viscous matter in the body, especially in the state of *zo 'f quwwat-i hazima*, or weak digestive power, thereby forming *khilt ghaliz* and *riah*, which accumulate in the urinary tract. These accumulations remain in the kidney for a long time, as the kidney has weak expulsive power, which is further diminished in the conditions such as *su-i mizaj kulliya, warm-i-har kulliya* and *qarah-i kulliya. Hararat* causes this morbid matter to transforms into gravel, which are either expelled through the kidneys or retained and converted into stones.

Razi writes in *Al-hawi* that the process of stone formation in any part of the body is secondary to the entanglement of *lesdar mawad* in the organs and the body's inability to expel the matter readily. This matter remains in the organs, and secondary deposition takes place over time. *Hararat* evaporates *rutoobat* from the matter and thereby forms a stone.

TYPES OF RENAL STONE

Urinary tract stones can be classified according to composition, location, size, aetiology, radiological characteristics and risk of recurrence.

Basically the renal stones can be divided into two major groups, primary stones and secondary stones.

Primary stone: These stones appear in healthy urinary tract without any inflammation. These are usually formed in the acidic urine. These stones usually consist of calcium oxalate, uric acid, urates, cystine, xanthine, or calcium carbonate.

Secondary stones: These are formed as the result of inflammation, in alkaline urine. Commonest types of stones are phosphate and mixed stones. Eighty percent of patients with Nephrolithiasis forms calcium stones, most of which are composed primarily of calcium oxalate or, less often, calcium phosphate. The other main types include uric acid, struvite, and cystine stones. A combination of different stone types may co-exist within a single stone.

1. Phosphate calculus: Majority of these stones are composed of calcium phosphate, though a few are composed of ammonium magnesium phosphate, known as 'triple phosphate'. Such calculus is usually smooth, soft and friable. It is usually dirty white in colour. This type of calculus usually occurs in infected urine and so is a secondary calculus. Urine is often alkaline. Such stone enlarges rapidly and gradually fills up pelvis and renal calyces to take up the shape of 'stag horn calculus '. As this stone gives little symptom due to its smooth surface, it enlarges rapidly. Triple phosphate usually results from liberation of ammonium carbonate from urea brought about by urea splitting organisms. While majority of such stones are made up of calcium phosphate, a few are made up of mixture of calcium phosphate and triple phosphate. On cut section it shows laminated appearance as the crystalloid are deposited in layers. These stones are usually radio-opaque as these contain calcium. But it is also due to its large size rather than density that it is radio-opaque.

2. Mixed stones: Phosphate stone may occur as covering of a primary stone. Such stones are known as 'mixed stones'. The primary stone is often the calcium oxalate stone. When the urine becomes infected deposits of phosphate occur on the rough surface of calcium oxalate stones. Such stones also occur in alkaline urine.

According to radiological classification, renal stones are radiopaque and radiolucent. Commonest radiolucent stone is uric acid stone. Less common radiolucent stones include xanthine and hypoxanthine stones. Radiopaque stones constitute the majority of renal stones. All calcium containing stones are radiopaque.

CLASSIFICATION OF STONES

Urinary stones can be classified according to size, location, X-ray characteristics, etiology of formation, composition and risk of recurrence.

Stone size: Stone size is usually given in one or two dimensions, and stratified into those measuring up to 5, 5-10, 10-20 and > 20 mm in largest diameter.

Stone location: Stones can be classified according to anatomical position: upper, middle or lower calyx; renal pelvis; upper, middle or distal ureter and urinary bladder.

X-ray characteristics: Stones can be classified according to plain X-ray appearance [kidney-ureter-bladder, KUB radiography] which varies according to mineral composition. Non-contrast enhanced computer tomography (NCCT) can be used to classify stones according to density, inner structure and composition, which can affect treatment decision. X-ray characteristics.

Radiopaque: Poor radiopacity Radiolucent Calcium oxalate dihydrate Calcium oxalate monohydrate calcium phosphates Magnesium, ammonium Apatite Cystine Phosphate, Uric acid Ammonium urate Xanthine, 2,8-dihydroxyadenine, Drug stones.

 Etiology of stone formation: Stones can be classified into those caused by, infectious or non-infectious causes (infectious and non-infectious stones) genetic defects or adverse drug effects (drug stones) Stones classified by etiology Non Infectious stones Infectious stones Genetic causes Drug stones Calcium oxalate Calcium phosphate Uric acid Magnesium ammonium phosphate Carbonate apatite Ammonium urate Cystine Xanthine 2,8-dihydroxyadenine

Types of renal calculus according to composition:

Oxalate calculus (calcium oxalate) Oxalate stones are irregular in shape and covered with sharp projections, which tend to cause bleeding. The surface of the calculus is discolored by altered blood. A calcium oxalate monohydrate stone is hard and radiodense.

Phosphate calculus: A phosphate calculus [calcium phosphate often with ammonium and magnesium phosphate (struvite)] is smooth and dirty white. It tends to grow in alkaline urine, especially when urea-splitting Proteus organisms are present. As a result, the calculus may enlarge to fill most of the collecting system, forming a stag horn calculus. Even a very large stag horn calculus may be clinically silent for years until it signals its presence by haematuria, urinary infection or renal failure. Because they are large, phosphate calculi are usually easy to see on radiographic films.

Uric acid and urate calculi: These are hard, smooth and often multiple. They vary from yellow to reddish brown and sometimes have an attractive, multifaceted appearance. Pure uric acid stones are radiolucent and appear on an excretory urogram as a filling defect, which can be mistaken for a transitional tumor of the upper urinary tract. The presence of uric acid stones is confirmed by CT. Most uric acid stones contain some calcium, so they cast a faint radiological shadow. In children, mixed stones of ammonium and sodium urate are sometimes found. They are yellow, soft and friable. They are radiolucent unless they are mixed with calcium salts.

Cystine calculus: These uncommon stones appear in the urinary tract of patients with a congenital error of metabolism that leads to cystinuria. Hexagonal, translucent, white crystals of cystine appear only in acidic urine. They are often multiple and may grow to form a cast of the collecting system. Pink or yellow when first removed, they change to a greenish color when exposed to air. Cystine stones are radio opaque because they contain sulphur, and they are very hard.

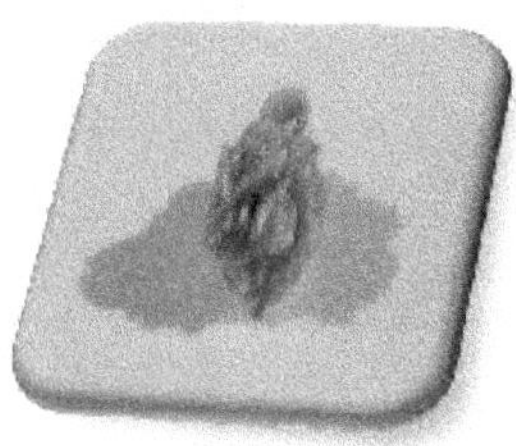

Calcium Oxalate Stone

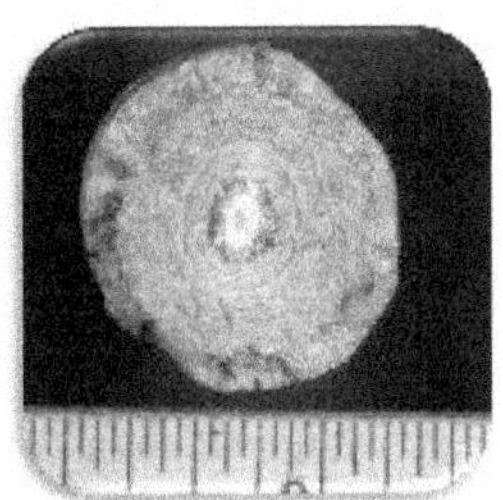

Calcium Oxalate with Uric acid nidus

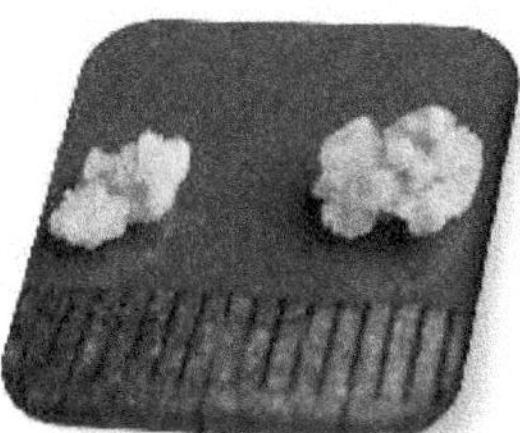

Calcium Phosphate Stone

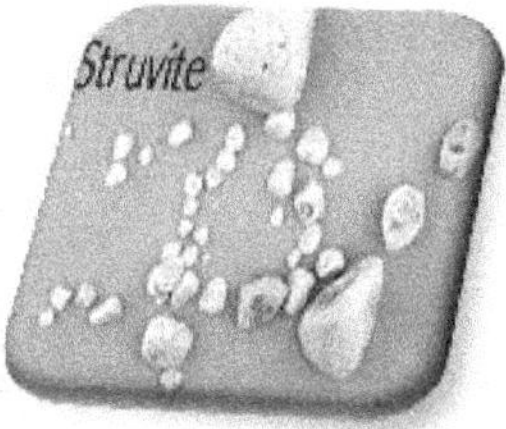

Struvite Stone

Clinical features

Renal calculi are common. Approximately 50% of patients present between the ages of 30 and 50 years. The male female ratio is 4:3.

Symptoms are variable and the diagnosis sometimes remains obscure until the stone is discovered on a radiograph.

Silent calculus/ Quiescent calculus

Urinary stones may occur anywhere in the urinary tract. Patients may occasionally be diagnosed with asymptomatic nephrolithiasis when a radiologic imaging study of the abdomen is performed for other purposes. They usually are asymptomatic in the renal pelvis or bladder, but they are a very common cause of symptomatic ureteral obstruction. The obstruction may be partial or complete. Calculi ≥ 7 mm are more likely to become impacted or to have a prolonged passage through the ureter. Even large staghorn calculi may cause no symptoms for long periods, during which time there is progressive destruction of the renal parenchyma. Uremia may be the first indication of bilateral calculi, although secondary infection usually produces symptoms first.

Pain

The clinical presentation is depends upon the size, position and type of the stone. Symptoms are usually produced when stones pass from the renal pelvis into the ureter. Pain is the leading symptom in 75% of people with urinary stones. Pain is the most common symptom and varies from a mild and barely noticeable ache to severe pain requiring parenteral analgesics. Common presentation is renal pain or ureteric colic.

Fixed renal pain is located posteriorly in the renal angle, anteriorly in the hypochondrium, or in both. It may be worse on movement, particularly on climbing stairs.

The referred pain associated with the renal colic usually originates from the flank and radiates to the front upper abdomen for kidney-related pain or radiates to the front toward the groin. Ureteric colic is an agonizing pain passing from the loin to the groin. Typically, it starts suddenly causing the patient to writhe to find comfort. Pain typically waxes and wanes in severity and develops in waves or paroxysms that are related to movement of the stone in the ureter and associated ureteral spasm. The site of obstruction from the stone generally determines the location of pain. Pain resulting from renal stones rarely lasts more than 8 hours in the absence of infection. There is no pyrexia, although the pulse rate rises because of the severe pain.

Ureteric colic is often caused by a stone entering the ureter but it may also occur when a stone becomes lodged in the pelviuretric junction. The severity of the colic is not related to the size of the stone. Ureteric colic may pass of with compensatory polyuria or passage of stone in the urine. Referred pain is rare and sometimes referred to all over abdomen. Such pain may simulate peptic ulcer or gall bladder disease. Sometime it may referred to opposite kidney, which is known as renorenal reflux.

Abdominal examination during an attack of ureteric colic there is rigidity of the lateral abdominal muscles.

Percussion over the kidney produces a stab of pain and there may be tenderness on gentle deep palpation.

Hydronephrosis or pyonephrosis leading to a palpable swelling in the loin is rare.
Hydronephrosis

Sometimes patient complaints of a lump in the loin and a dull ache, which may be due to hydronephrosis caused by renal stones.

Haematuria

Haematuria is sometimes a leading symptom of stone disease and occasionally the only one. As a rule, the amount of bleeding is small. Often, microscopic Haematuria and less commonly, gross haematuria are associated with the patient with acute Nephrolithiasis. **Pyuria:** Infection is likely in the presence of stones and is particularly dangerous when the kidney is obstructed. As pressure builds in the dilated collecting system, organisms are injected into the circulation and a life-threatening septicaemia can quickly develop. The mechanical effect of stones irritating the urothelium may cause Pyuria even in the absence of infection.

Dysuria, Difficulty in passing urine, Burning Micturation, Frequency of Micturation, Heaviness in flank, Feeling of something hanging in Flank during sleep in prone position, Stabbing pain, Pain in scrotum and leg of affected side. During movement of stone from flank to Groin pain is reffered from flank to groin, Nausea and vomiting.

Renal stones are common, may be clinically silent even when large. They are usually visible on a plain abdominal radiograph, may be radiolucent when composed of uric acid. Ureteric colic is a pattern of severe exacerbation on a background of continuing pain. It radiates to the groin, penis, scrotum or labium as the stone progresses down the ureter. The severity of pain is not related to the size of the stone. The pain is almost invariably associated with haematuria. There may be few physical signs.

Physical sign

i) **Tenderness**: Mostly present at the renal angle posteriorly, this angle is between the lower border of 12th rib & the lateral border of the erector spinae muscles. Anteriorly such tenderness may be elicited about a inch below and medial to the tip of the 9th costal cartilage, which is known as the renal point. Tenderness is more constant feature when renal calculus is associated with infection.

ii) **Muscle rigidity** over the kidney may be found in a few cases. Rebound tenderness anteriorly can also be elicited, particularly if acute infection is associated with.

iii) **Swelling in the flank** when there is hydronephrosis or pyonephrosis associated with renal calculus.

The characteristics of a renal swelling are:

(a) It is oval or reniform in shape.

(b) The swelling is almost fixed and cannot be moved as it is a retroperitoneal swelling.

(c) A kidney lump is ballotable.

(d) The swelling slightly moves up and down with respiration, but much less than a liver swelling.

(e) Fingers can be insinuated between the lump and the costal margin (which is not possible in splenic or liver swelling).

(f) A band of resonance can be elicited anteriorly on percussion, due to presence of colon, duodenum and coils of small intestine in front of the kidney according to the side (but such resonance is absent in splenic and liver swellings).

(iv) **Abdominal distension** and diminished peristalsis may accompany ureteric colic.

In Unani system of Medicine the renal calculus is named as *"Hasat-e-Kulliya"*. Ancient literatures described broadly the pathology, manifestations and treatment of *Hasat-e-kulliya*. Signs, Symptoms, and Diagnosis In Unani medicine, the *atībbā'* (physician) valuates *nabz* (pulse), *baul* (urine), and *barāz* (stools) in order to diagnose disease, and when urolithiasis is suspected, the urine is carefully examined to make the final diagnosis. Patients are advised to collect urine overnight in a clean container that must be protected from contaminants. On the following day, the urine is discarded without disturbing any sediment in the container. Red or yellow sediments are diagnostic of urinary stones or gravel. When urine transforms from thick and viscous to clear and watery, the morbid matter is accumulating in the kidneys and thereby causing stone formation. When black-colored urine appears in the absence of systemic disease or pain in the lumbar region accompanied with abdominal colic, then kidney stones are thought to have formed. If the pain radiates from the loin towards the pubic area, it is assumed that the calculi are descending in the ureter. Reduced severity of pain in the lumbar region suggests that the renal calculi have reached the bladder. Signs and symptoms of bladder calculi are dysuria, incomplete voiding of urine, irritation at the root of the urethra, and pruritis over the penis, which compels the patients to rub his hands over the pubic region. The gravel and sediments of bladder calculi are muddy or white.

According to *Ibn Sīnā*, renal calculi are soft, small, and usually red in colour, whereas bladder calculi are hard, large, and sandy white in colour. Renal calculi cause heaviness in the lumbar region when the intestines are full. The colour of urine will be yellow-red. Signs and symptoms of urinary calculi are presence of sediments in the urine, lower back pain, numbness in the legs, and dysuria. The sediments may be yellow, red, or brown, and may resemble pomegranate seeds. Urinary disturbance accompanied by pain in the loin region during micturation, nausea and constipation suggests that calculi are present in both kidneys.

Rufus narrated that if a person is passing black urine without any disease along with pain or without pain, it confirms that after a time period he will develop renal stone especially in elderly person, so once should use diuretics (*mudir bol)* as early as possible. Further he cited that the use of black and offensive clay added with sulphur *(gandhak)* can act as good antiurolithiatic agent.

Iristatalis has narrated that when a person having calculi is passing crystals (reeg) in urine, it predict that the calculi is soft and fragile in nature. So it can be breakdown and excreted with the help of drugs easily while as if the urine of person having calculi is very clear is denoting that the calculi is very hard and unfragiable in nature/ unable to breakdown.

Yahoodi citated that person who were passing more amount of salt in their urine are more prone to develop renal calculi.

Mohaammed bin zakariya razi said that I had observed that children had more amount of salt in their urine.

Ahran citated that the color of bladder calculi will be white while as the color of renal calculi will be red. He further said that adults always develop renal calculi and children always develop bladder calculi.

Ibn Sarabiyun narrated that if the calculi is impacted in a particular area of kidney then pain will be over that particular area. If the stone is moving then in first phase patient will be calm and relax as well as in second phase there will be severe pain.

Ali bin Zain has quoted that renal calculi should be treated with drugs having hot temperament (*advia harra*) so that the drug will breakdown the calculi, but the chosen drug should not have excessive hot temperament by which they can cause dryness which may increase stiffness in consistency of calculi.

Presentation and Differential Diagnosis:

Urolithiasis should always be considered in the differential diagnosis of abdominal pain. The classical presentation of renal colic is excruciating unilateral flank or lower abdominal pain of sudden onset that is not related to any precipitating event and is not relieved by postural changes or non-narcotic medications. With the exception of nausea and vomiting secondary to stimulation of the celiac plexus, gastrointestinal symptoms are usually absent. The pain of renal colic often begins as vague flank pain. Patients frequently dismiss this pain until it evolves into waves of severe pain. It is generally believed that a stone must at least partially obstruct the Ureter to cause pain. The pain is commonly referred to the lower abdomen and to the ipsilateral groin. As the stone progresses down the Ureter, the pain tends to migrate caudally and medially. Distal ureteral stones may be manifested by bladder instability, urinary frequency, dysuria and/or pain radiating to the tip of the penis, or the labia or vulva. Increasingly, however, calculi are encountered in asymptomatic patients and are found incidentally on imaging studies or during the evaluation of microhematuria. Symptoms similar to those of renal colic can be caused by non-calculus conditions.

In women, gynecological problems that must be considered, include ovarian torsion, ovarian cyst and ectopic pregnancy.

In men, symptoms of testicular processes, such as a tumor, epididymitis or prostatitis, may mimic the symptoms of distal ureteral stones.

Other general causes of abdominal pain, such as appendicitis, cholecystitis, diverticulitis, colitis, constipation, hernias or even arterial aneurysms, may elicit similar discomfort.

Symptoms mimicking those of urolithiasis also occur with urologic lesions such as congenital ureteropelvic junction obstruction, renal or ureteral tumors, and other causes of ureteral obstruction.

COMPLICATION

Effect of the stone: The size and position of the stone usually govern the development of secondary pathologic changes in the urinary tract.

SAME KIDNEY

Obstruction

• A stone lodged at the ureteropelvic junction or in the ureter may cause hydronephrosis if the obstruction is intermittent or incomplete.

• When the obstruction is complete it may slowly destroy the kidney.

Infection

This is a common complication due to stasis of urine caused by the stone and it also acts like a foreign body, such infection may cause pyelitis, pyelonephritis, pelvinephric adhesion and even pelvinephric abscess. When infection is superimposed with hydronephrosis, pyonephrosis may result. The Epithelium of the pelvis and calyces in relation to the stone gradually loses luster becomes rough and thickened, parenchymal ischemia may be caused by local pressure due to stone. Sometimes due to presence of stone the lining epithelium of the pelvis may undergo metaplasia (from normal transitional variety to squamous variety) which may initiate malignancy of epidermoid nature (epithelioma).

OPPOSITE KIDNEY

i. Compensatory hypertrophy may occur when the affected kidney has lost function due to complete obstruction with stone.

ii. Stone formation may be bilateral.

iii. Infection of the opposite kidney may result from ascending infection from the urinary bladder when urine becomes infected due to presence of stone.

iv. Calculus anuria- reflex cessation of function of the opposite kidney occurs due to reno-renal reflex caused by complete obstruction of the affected kidney with calculus.

Kidney stones and chronic kidney disease (CKD) were reported in 5% and 13% of the adult population respectively. CKD is a complication of kidney stones as a result of rare hereditary disorders. Kidney stones may be associated with complications such as infection, acute renal failure (due to obstructive uropathy) and chronic kidney damage. The prevalence of the end-stage renal disease (ESRD) due to kidney stones among patients who start maintenance haemodialysis was approximately 3.2%. Infectious stones are the most frequent cause of urolithiasis associated ESRD, especially in bilateral developing of stag horn stones. Extensive stone development has been observed with uric acid, calcium oxalate or cystine stones. The potential risk of degradation of renal function justifies the etiological investigation of all lithiasis associated pathologies. Haemodialysis and recurrent infections are seen in patients with renal stones. Stone can cause the obstruction, secondary infection, pyonephrosis, renal failure, Ureteral stricture, Urine extravasation, Perinephric abscess and Xanthogranulomatous pyelonephritis.

Diagnosis

Patients with urinary stones usually present with loin pain, vomiting, and sometime fever but may also be asymptomatic. The diagnosis of nephrolithiasis is initially suspected by the clinical presentation.

According to presence of stones the symptoms are

Relationship of Stone Location to Symptoms

Stone location	Common symptoms
Kidney	Vague flank pain, haematuria
Proximal ureter	Renal colic, flank pain, upper abdominal pain
Middle ureter	Renal colic, anterior abdominal pain, flank pain
Distal ureter	Renal colic, dysuria, urinary frequency, anterior abdominal pain, flank pain

Special investigations:

1 Blood examination

This hardly reveals any specific abnormality, but an increased white blood cell count may be seen when associated with infection. Anaemia may be found if renal function is not adequate.

Renal function must be assessed by estimating blood urea and creatinine.

If serum proteins are decreased but total calcium is normal, an increase in ionised calcium is indicated Hypercalcaemia with hypophosphataemia strongly suggests primary hyperparathyroidism, though normal serum phosphate is found in 60% of patients. Estimation of serum chloride concentration is helpful in this respect as when it is above 102 mEq/L it is a case of hyperparathyroidism and when it is below this figure it may be due to hypercalcaemia from other causes. Serum hypercalcaemia is very much associated with calculus disease, though it is commonly associated with osteolytic and disseminated malignant diseases e.g. cancers of the breast, lungs, multiple myeloma, leukaemia etc. It is also seen in sarcoidosis. But these conditions rarely cause renal stones. Elevated serum uric acid level is found in 50% of uric acid stone carriers.

2 Urinalysis

(i) **Physical examination** may show smoky urine due to slight haematuria or opalescent due to presence of pus.

(ii) **Chemical examination** may show presence of protein due to haematuria and blood in the urine. If pH of the urine is higher than 7.6, presence of urea-splitting organisms is assured. This also denotes that the stone is probably of triple phosphate Consistently low pH is a common cause of formation of uric acid calculi A simple chemical test for cystine may be performed by making the urine alkaline with ammonium hydroxide and then 2 ml of 5% sodium cyanide is added and the urine is allowed to stand for 5 minutes A few drops of fresh 5% sodium nitroprusside is added. A deep purplish-red colour means cystinuria.

(iii) **Microscopic examination of urine** may show R.B.C., pus cells and casts. Different crystals may be seen in the sediment to give a clue as to the type of stone present Uric acid and cystine crystals may be precipitated by adding a few drops of glacial acetic acid, which lowers the urinary pH to about 4.The test tube of urine is then

> refrigerated. Uric acid crystals are shown amber-brown, whereas cystine crystals look like benzene rings.
>
> (iv) **Bacteriological** examination of urine is highly important including culture and sensitivity tests.
>
> (v) **Renal function tests** should always be performed in calculus cases. The PSP may be normal even in presence of bilateral staghorn calculi. But it may be depressed to 2/3 rds of normal in acute obstruction at the ureteropelvic junction

With the exception of renal and scrotal masses or tenderness, a palpable bladder or an abnormal prostate on digital rectal examination, urological conditions are most likely to be diagnosed from the history or by investigations.

Urine Dipsticks (Multistix, Labstix) are a convenient way to screen urine for blood, protein or nitrites. When the urine is macroscopically clear and negative on dipstick testing, microscopy and culture of a midstream clean-catch specimen are usually negative.

The presence of protein and nitrites (produced by organisms in the urine) indicates the likelihood of infection. Some dipsticks also give an indication of the pH and specific gravity of the urine.

Microscopic haematuria may be detected by dipstick testing in a routine health check. A substantial haemorrhage imparts a red or brownish tinge to the urine (macroscopic haematuria) and the patient may pass clots. False-positive stick tests and the discoloured urine caused by beetroot and some drugs (e.g. Dindevan (phenindione), Pyridium (phenazopyridine) and Furadantin (nitrofurantoin)) are distinguishable by the absence of red blood cells on urinary microscopy

Microscopy confirms the presence of white and red blood cells in the urine, and bacteria may also be visible. Protein casts suggest disease of the renal parenchyma, as doe's red cell dysmorphia seen on phase contrast microscopy. Schistosoma ova have a typical appearance, and vegetable or meat fibres may be present if there is a fistula connecting the bowel with the urinary tract.

Bacteriological culture of a clean-catch midstream specimen of the urine is the standard means of identifying urinary pathogens. Organisms at a level of >105 /mL is deemed to indicate the presence of infection rather than contamination of the urine by bacteria. If there are pus cells in the urine but there is no growth on the routine culture media (sterile pyuria), it is worth testing for more fastidious organisms. The centrifuged sediment of multiple early-morning urine specimens are cultured on Löwenstein–Jensen medium to detect urinary tract tuberculosis. Chlamydia is another common urinary pathogen that will not be detected on routine culture.

Biochemical examination for electrolytes, glucose, bilirubin, haemoglobin and myoglobin is essential to detect abnormal amounts of these substances in the urine. Analysis of a 24-hour specimen of urine will quantify the rate of loss, and is especially useful in the investigation of calculus disease caused by abnormal excretion of calcium, oxalate, uric acid and other products of metabolism

Microscopic, cytological, bacteriological and biochemical examination of urine

■ Abnormalities found on Multistik testing of the urine should be confirmed by microscopy and culture

■ More than 105 organisms per mL of urine is deemed to indicate a significant urinary infection

■ Cytological examination of the urine will usually detect a poorly differentiated transitional cell tumour

Tests of renal function

■ Elevated blood urea and serum creatinine levels usually indicate a significant impairment of renal function

■More sophisticated renal assessment is required to quantify the functional deficit

3. Radiography

A. STRAIGHT X-RAY:

A plain abdominal x-ray showing the kidneys, ureters and bladder (the KUB) is a simple and useful test. Before taking straight X-ray for KUB region (both kidneys, ureters and bladder), the bowels must be made empty by giving laxative

Straight X-ray shows At least 90% of renal stones are radio-opaque and are easily branched renal calculus in right kidney. Visible in a plane film of KUB region unless they are very small or overlie bones. A staghom calculus can be easily diagnosed and there is no confusion with other radioopaque shadows. It is necessary to differentiate renal stone from other structures and pathologies which may produce radio-opaque shadow on straight X-ray similar to a renal calculus.

These structures and pathologies are as follows :

(i) Phleboliths.

(ii) Ossified tip of the 12th rib.

(iii) A calcified lumbar or mesenteric lymph nodes.

(iv) Gallstones.

(v) A chip fracture of the transverse process of a lumbar vertebra.

(vi) A calcified tuberculous lesion of the kidney.

(vii) A calcified suprarenal gland.

(viii) A few drugs e.g. fersolate or foreign bodies in the G.I. tract.

The characteristic features of renal stone are:

(a) Exposures are made during full inspiration and full expiration. If the opaque material moves with the kidney as measured from the lower pole of the kidney, it is probably a renal stone.

(b) Renal stone is usually equal in density (whereas gallstones are usually ring shaped with a radiolucent centre).

(c) In a doubtful case a lateral radiograph should be taken. If the opaque material is seen in front of the bodies of the vertebrae, it is not a renal stone. A renal stone is superimposed on the bodies of the vertebrae.

Preparation of the patient:

Enema/bowel wash/laxative is given on the previous day and the patient is asked to fast in order to reduce the bowel gas shadows in X-ray.

♦ High penetration X-ray is taken in supine position which covers pubic symphysis and lower two ribs.

♦ **interpreting the film**:

 a. First bony parts are looked for, i.e. the hip, pelvis, lumbar vertebrae for fractures, scoliosis, spina bifida, secondaries in the spine.

b. Kidney shadow: Kidney shadows are visualised in plain X-ray KUB due to difference in the density between kidney (high vascularity) and perinephric fat (low vascularity). Findings noted are size, location, calcification and stones. In children, perinephric fat is absent and so kidney shadows are not visualised.

c. Psoas shadow: It is visualised well in normal KUB.

Psoas shadow is obliterated in:

In enlarged kidney

In scoliosis due to infl ammatory or infi ltrative causes

In malignancy

Tuberculous spine with cold abscess (psoas abscess)

Splenic injury—in left sided shadow

Retroperitoneal tumours

d. Ureteric line: It is looked for any radio-opaque shadow (ureteric stone). It runs along the tips of the transverse processes of the lumbar vertebrae, crosses the sacroiliac joints and reaches up to a point medial to the ischial spine.

e. Bladder, prostate and urethral areas are visualised for any lesion.

Intravenous urography (urography)

Excretion renography has been a mainstay of urological investigation since the introduction of intravenous contrast media in the 1930s. These are organic chemicals to which iodine atoms are attached to absorb x-rays. When such a chemical is injected intravenously, it is filtered from the blood by the glomeruli and does not undergo tubular absorption. As a result, it rapidly passes through the renal parenchyma into the urine, which it renders radio-opaque. Although intravenous urography (IVU) gives excellent images of the urinary tract (Figure 74.3), its use should be restricted because in a few patients the iodine in the contrast medium may cause an anaphylactic reaction. Patients with a history of allergy, atopy and eczema are particularly vulnerable, but severe reactions may occur without warning. Less invasive and dangerous imaging techniques are clearly to be preferred if they are able to give comparable diagnostic information.

Intravenous urography

- IVU can cause a dangerous hypersensitivity reaction in a small number of patients

Preparation

A laxative will clear faeces that might otherwise obscure details of urinary tract anatomy. Modest fluid restriction is permissible, but dehydration is dangerous because it may precipitate acute renal failure.

Technique

The patient is observed carefully while the first few drops of contrast medium (Urografin or Niopam 370) are injected. The earliest films show the renal parenchyma opacified by contrast medium – the nephrogram phase. A delayed nephrogram on one side indicates unilateral functional impairment. Distortion of the renal outline or failure of part of the kidney to function suggests a space-occupying lesion. After a few minutes, the contrast is excreted into the collecting system, opacifying the calyces and the renal pelvis. Later films show the ureters and, at the end of the study, the patient is asked to pass urine and a final film is taken to show details of the bladder area. It is important to bear in mind that the static images of IVU provide only snapshots of dynamic events in the urinary tract. The appearance of a normal ureter changes as peristaltic waves of contraction pass along it. IVU is particularly valuable to demonstrate tumours and calculi within the urinary tract, which are sometimes difficult to see on ultrasonography. It may also be useful to show details of abnormal anatomy that are difficult to interpret on an ultrasonogram. As ultrasonography and other forms of scanning have become more sophisticated, the indications for the urogram are fewer and it may eventually fall into disuse. Obstruction to the upper urinary tract interferes with transport of contrast medium into the urine, which will show up as a non-functioning kidney on the standard urogram films. In these circumstances, a further x-ray taken many hours after injection of the contrast medium may show hazy opacification of a dilated system. Distortion of the calyces or the renal outline can equally be caused by a tumour or by harmless simple cysts. In each of these cases, more information can be obtained from ultrasonography or computed tomography (CT).

Retrograde ureteropyelography (synonym: retrograde ureterogram)

A ureteric catheter is passed into the ureteric orifice through a cystoscope.Contrast medium injected through the catheter will demonstrate the anatomy of the upper urinary tract. This is particularly useful if there is doubt about an intraluminal lesion or if renal function is deficient (before surgery for pelviureteric junction obstruction, for instance). When a transitional tumour is found, it can be sampled by aspiration of urine from the upper tract or by brush biopsy. Retrograde ureteropyelography is possible under topical urethral anaesthesia using a flexible cystoscope. Introducing infection into a poorly draining part of the system carries a serious risk of septicaemia. If there is to be any delay in correcting the blockage surgically, facilities must be available to decompress the kidney by retrograde stenting or percutaneous nephrostomy.

Antegrade pyelography

Percutaneous puncture of a dilated renal collecting system is reasonably simple. The most common indication is the placement of a nephrostomy tube to drain an obstructed infected kidney or to provide access for percutaneous nephrolithotomy. Antegrade pyelography – in which contrast medium is introduced through the nephrostomy – can be helpful when retrograde studies are prevented by obstruction at the extreme lower end of the ureter

Digital subtraction arteriography Refinements in radiological imaging have now almost eliminated the need for translumbar aortography. Satisfactory imaging of the renal vessels can be achieved by digital subtraction angiography after intravenous injection of contrast medium. More precise information can be obtained by intra-arterial injection through a fine catheter inserted into the femoral artery using the Seldinger technique. Arteriography is now rarely used to demonstrate tumour vasculature in a hypernephroma (Figure 74.6), but a flush venogram is useful when CT suggests tumour invasion of the renal vein and vena cava.

Cystography

Cystography is now most commonly a component of videourodynamic assessment (see Chapter 76). Its role in assessing ureteric reflux in children has been largely superseded by radioisotope scanning and dynamic ultrasonography. Urethrography Ascending urethrography is valuable to demonstrate the extent of a urethral stricture (Figure 74.7) and the presence of false passages and diverticula associated with it. A urethrogram can be used to assess the extent of urethral trauma, but there is a serious danger that contrast medium may pass into the circulation. Lipiodol carries the danger of fat embolus and should never be used, and death has followed the use of barium emulsion. Umbradil viscous V is a radio-opaque water-soluble gel that contains the local anaesthetic lignocaine. It can be injected gently and safely using Knutsson's apparatus even if the urothelium is breached. Venography Extension of a renal carcinoma from the renal vein into the vena cava can usually be demonstrated by ultrasound or CT, but venography was used for this purpose.

Ultrasonography

Ultrasonography is perhaps the imaging technique most widely used in urology. Kidney size, the thickness of its cortex and the presence and degree of hydronephrosis can be measured with great accuracy. Intrarenal masses can be diagnosed as smooth walled and fluid filled (simple cysts) or solid and complex (possible tumours). Stones produce a bright ultrasonic reflection and cast an acoustic shadow. The volume of urine in the bladder before and after micturition can be calculated, and even tiny filling defects within it detected. Scrotal contents can be displayed in great detail. The prostate is accessible by the transrectal route. Only the lower ureter resists effective investigation by transabdominal ultrasonography because of its small calibre and its proximity to the large bones of the pelvis and spine.

Ultrasonography

■ Ultrasound scanning provides broadly similar anatomical information to an intravenous urogram but without the risks.

Transrectal ultrasonography

This has become a routine component of the investigation of suspected carcinoma of the prostate. Most commonly, suspicion has arisen because the level of prostate-specific antigen is raised or there is an abnormality of the texture or outline of the prostate on digital rectal examination. The features of carcinoma or benign enlargement of the prostate, although not absolutely specific, are sufficiently well recognised to allow an experienced ultrasonographer to identify promising sites for transrectal fine needle biopsy. Computed tomography CT is particularly useful to assess structures in the retro peritoneum.

In renal carcinoma it will show:

• The size and site of the tumour and the degree of invasion of adjacent tissue;

• The presence of enlarged lymph nodes at the renal hilum;

• Invasion of the renal vein and vena cava.

CT is of crucial importance in the initial staging and follow up of men with testicular cancer, in whom the presence of retroperitoneal lymph node masses features in advanced disease. It has also been used to stage bladder and prostate cancer, but its value is less clear cut in these diseases. Non-contrast CT is also used routinely in the diagnosis of urinary calculi. Magnetic resonance imaging and positron emission tomography. These technologies give information about the function of organs as well as detailed structural images. As they become more widely available, they are replacing many of the routine imaging techniques.

Radioisotope scanning

Radioisotope scanning is used to obtain information about function in individual renal units. Diethyltriaminepentaacetic acid (DTPA) is filtered by the glomeruli and not absorbed by the tubules. Using a gamma camera, DTPA labelled with technetium-99m can be followed during its transit through individual kidneys to give a dynamic representation of renal function. A 99mTc-DTPA scan is particularly useful to prove that collecting system dilatation is caused by obstruction.

Ascending urethrogram demonstrating a tight stricture in the bulbar urethra. Above the stricture the contrast outlines the prostatic urethra and bladder. A calculus in the kidney casts an acoustic shadow (courtesy of Dr Matthew Matson).

Computed tomography showing renal cell carcinoma of the right kidney.

Anuria: a diuretic like frusemide (furosemide).

Other substances (dimercaptosuccinic acid (DMSA), mercaptoacetylglycine (MAG-3) and sodium orthoiodohippurate (Hippuran)) labelled with suitable radioactive isotopes have similarly been used to investigate renal function. Isotope bone scanning is fundamental to the staging of kidney and prostate cancers, which typically metastasise to the skeleton. Endoscopy Visual inspection of the lower urinary tract has been possible since 1877, when Nitze invented his cystoscope. A leap forward in urological endoscopy came with the introduction by Hopkins of the rod lens telescope and fibreoptic illumination. This allowed development of a family of endoscopes, which allow the urologist to visualise the upper and lower urinary tracts for diagnosis and therapy. Finally, in the early 1980s, the small calibre flexible fibrescopic cystoscope was introduced. This allows simple diagnostic cystourethroscopy, bladder biopsy and retrograde ureterography to be performed under topical urethral anaesthesia with minimal discomfort to the patient.

PREVENTION:

Dietary Changes to Help Prevent Kidney Stones

People can help prevent kidney stones by making changes in fluid intake and depending on the type of kidney stone, changes in consumption of sodium, animal protein, calcium and oxalate.

Drinking enough fluids each day is the best way to help prevent most types of kidney stones. Health care providers recommend that a person drink 2 to 3 litres of fluid a day. People with cystine stones may need to drink even more. Though water is best, other fluids may also help prevent kidney stones, such as citrus drinks.

Recommendations based on the specific type of kidney stone include the following

Calcium Oxalate Stones

• reducing sodium

• reducing animal protein, such as meat, eggs, and fish

• getting enough calcium from food or taking calcium supplements with food

• avoiding foods high in oxalate, such as spinach, rhubarb, nuts, and wheat bran

Calcium Phosphate Stones

• reducing sodium

• reducing animal protein

• getting enough calcium from food or taking calcium supplements with food

Uric Acid Stones

• limiting animal protein.

USOOL ILAJ

Unani Modalities for the Management of Renal Calculus

The management of diseases depends upon the pathology involved in the disease process. In the Unani system of Medicine goal for the treatment for renal calculi is to make morbid and abnormal humours easily out of the body through the excretory system.

Following Principles are implicated in the Management of Renal Calculus

Removal of underlying causes

Through proper history, examinations, and investigations.

Tanqiya mawad (cleansing of morbid matter) and *tadeel mizaj.*

The *tanqiye mawad* of this disease through the drugs which has the following properties like *muhallil-e-awram* (Anti-inflammatory), *mulattif* (deobstruent), *mufattit hissat* (lithotriptic), *mudire-bol* (diuretic) and *Muqawwi gurda.*

To correct indigestion and constipation: If the patient is having these problems.

In Unani System of Medicine, the Management of any Diseases is Laid down on the Following Parameters

- ✓ Dietotherapy
- ✓ Regimental therapy
- ✓ Pharmacotherapy
- ✓ Surgery

However, the first treatment preference is diet therapy, regimental therapy, followed by pharmacotherapy and surgery only if required.

Dietotherapy

Diet therapy has an essential role in the prevention of disease rather than its control. Unani physicians give prime importance to diet and the state of digestion in a person, in both health and disease. According to *Buqrat* (Hippocrate), the quality (*Kaifiyat*) and quantity (*Kammiyat*) of diet, and the importance of a balanced diet concerning the occurrence of the disease are important factors. Specific dietary regimens are recommended while treating patients according to their temperament. Proper foods are assumed to produce good humours (*Akhlat Saliha*) while odd ones produce bad humours (*Akhlat Radiyya*). Thus, the *humoral* imbalance can be corrected by medication coupled with proper diet i.e diet plays a vital role in the management of disease.

Diet Recommended

• *Aab-e-Naryl* (coconut water), carrot, chicken

• Goats heart (*qalb-e-ghenam*) and sparrow (*Asaafeer*).

Diet Restricted High oxalate diet like *Amlah*, tomato, cashew nuts, pumpkin, spinach, amaranth leaves, mushrooms, cauliflower, brinjal etc.

Regimental Therapy

The basic aim of *Ilaj bil-Tadbeer* is to change the consistency (soft) of morbid matter through the following regimental therapies such as:

• Purgation (*Mushilat*)

• Enema (*Huqna*)

• Venesection (*Fasd*)

• Sitz bath (*Abzan*)

Purgation: Mild purgatives like *Anjeer* (Ficus Carica), *Maghze-Amaltas* (Cassia fistula), *Asl-us-soos* (*Glycyrrhiza glabra*)

Huqna (Enema*):* Huqna of *Mulayyin* and *Muzliq* (Laxative and Emollient) like *Tukhm-e-Katan* (Linum usitatissimum), *Tukhm-e-Khatami* (Althea Officinalis)

Fasd (venesection): *Rag-e-Basaleeq* (Baselic vein).

Aabzan (Sitz bath): Decoction containing *murakhkhi* and *musakkin* drugs such as *Khatmi, Shibt, Hulba, Baboona, Khurfah and Banafasha.*

Pharmacotherapy Drugs can be used which has the following properties like anti-inflammatory, deobstruent, lithotriptic, and diuretics for the treatment of renal calculus.

Single drugs

There are many single drugs which can be used as shown in the following table.

S. No.	Drug name	Botanical name	Medicinal uses
1	*Habb-ul-Qilt*	Dolio biflorus	Lithotriptics, mulattif, diuretic
2	*Khar-e- khasak*	Tribulus terrestris	Diuretic, anti-inflammatory, lithotriptic
3	*Habb-e-Kaaknaj*	Physalis alkekengi	Diuretic, lithotriptics
4	*Aaloo balu*	Prunus cerasus	Anti-inflammatory, lithotripti
5	*Shora qalmi*	Potassium nitrate	Diuretic
6	*Sange sarmahi*	Fish stone	Lithotriptic
7	*Jawakhar*	Potassium carbonates	Lithotriptic, diuretic
8	*Hajrul yahood*	Lapis judaicus	Lithotriptic

| 9 | . *Aqrab sokhta* | Burnt scorpion | Lithotriptic |
| 10 | . *Tukhme kharpaza* | Cucumis melo linn | Diuretic, lithotriptic, mulattif |

Compound drug used for *hasat-e-kulliya.*

S. No	Compound name	Therapeutic action
1.	*Majoon Sangesarmahi*	Lithotriptic
2.	*Sharbate Aaloo balu*	Lithotriptic
3.	*Sharbate bazoori moatadil*	Diuretic
4.	*Qurse Kaknaj*	Lithotriptic,
5.	*Majoon-e-Ibn-e-Sarafiyun*	Lithotriptic,
6.	*Majoon Aqrab*	Lithotriptic,
7.	*Kushta Hajr-ul Yahood*	Lithotriptic,
8.	*Jawarish Zarooni Ambari*	Muqawwiye gurda
9.	*Majoon Hajr-ul-yahood*	Lithotriptic,
10	*Majoon kaaknaj*	Lithotriptic,

According to *Rufus* if a person is passing black urine without any disease along with pain or without pain, it confirms that after a time period he will develop renal stone especially in elderly person, so once should use (diuretics) *mudir bol* as early as possible. Further he cited that the use of black and offensive clay added with *gandhak* (sulphur) can act as good antiurolithiatic agent. *Ali bin Zain* has quoted that renal calculi should be treated with drugs having hot temperament *(advia harra)* so that the drug will breakdown the calculi, but the chosen drug should not have excessive hot temperament by which they can cause dryness which may increase stiffness in consistency of calculi.

Preventive Measures

• Fluid: Intake should be 3-4 lit/day and output 2 lit/ day at least. Intake is distributed throughout the day

• Sodium: Restrict intake • Protein: Moderate, not high

• Calcium: Avoid supplements from meal, avoidance of milk, cheese

• Oxalate: Avoid foods rich in oxalate e.g., spinach, rhubarb, etc.

According to Unani physician's line of treatment of *Hasat-e-Kulliya* is

● Remove the *Asbabe Maddi* (causative material),

● Use of *Mufattite Hasat advia* (lithotriptic drugs) and

● Use of *Mudir Bol advia* (diuretics drugs).

Accumulation of morbid matter can be removed by *Mudir bol advia* through urinary system, further it can be avoided by restriction of diets (*ghaleez aghzia*), which are responsible for the formation of *hasat* e.g. concentrated milk, paneer and meat (old camel, old bull, old goat), roasted meat, fish meat and *sangeen roti* (feteeri, leshdar maida) etc. The principles of management of Renal calculi in Unani medicine is mainly through diuretic and lithotriptic (crushing) drugs to make morbid and abnormal *humors* easily extractible from the body mainly through the excretory system.

Drugs Beneficial in Urolithiasis

In *Kitabul Kulliyāt, Ibn Rushd* describes the statements of many *atibbā* that, the drugs used as *mufattit i hissāt* (lithotryptic) must have mild degree of *harārat* because severe degree of *hararat* makes substances harder, such as the *harārat-i gharībā* (abnormal heat) responsible for the formation of renal stones. Hence the amount of *harārat* in the drugs used as lithotryptic must be less than that required for the formation of stones.

The principle used is, any substance or morbid matter which is under the influence of *harārat* (hot) and *yabusat* (dry) can be correct by *burūdat* (cold) and *rutubāt* (moist). Hence the temperament of drugs to be used for the treatment of urolithiasis must be less hot comparatively. These mild degree drugs bring equilibrium in the morbid matter or substance and the *harārat-i gharīziyā* expels them out of the body. The drugs beneficial are *halyun, chana* and *bādām* etc. It is also possible that these drugs act due to their constituents and their characteristic features. Drugs which are used to expel the urinary stones must be *talkh* (bitter) in taste, not very hot and have the property of *taqtī* (cutting, making into small bits). Drugs used for bladder calculi must be slightly hotter than those used for renal calculi. However few drugs are used which act because of their *mufattit* (lithotryptic) property and not because of hot or cold temperament. There are some drugs which are useful in renal calculi than in bladder calculi such has *hajrul yahūd*. Few drugs are beneficial in both bladder and renal calculi such as *Majoon aqrab*. Some drugs do not have the property of *nuzj*, but a few are *mufattit* as well as have the property of *nuzj* like *habbul qil qil*. *Mudir i baul* (diuretic) drugs also have mild degree of *harārat*, which helps the kidneys to absorb the liquid matter. All those drugs which are *tez* act as diuretics such as *Karafs, Bādiyān, dūqū* etc.

Surgery

Masīhī states, "In case of obstruction of urine due to calculus and when no other option is available except for surgery, bladder calculus can be removed by applying perineal incision. Procedure is called perineal cystolithotomy. *Abū al-Qāsim al-Zaharāwī* (936-1013 AD) in his medical encyclopedia *"Altasriyf liman ajiza anialta lify"* has described over 200 surgical instruments with illustrations and method of their manufacture. In urology, he described the drilling on urethral stones and the operation of vaginal lithotomy. *Ibn Sīnā* introduced the technique of instillation of medication into the urethra.

MANAGMNT OF RENAL SONE ACCORDING TO ALTERNATIVE THERAPY

Treatment of nephrolithiasis involves emergency management of renal (ureteral) colic, including surgical interventions where indicated, and medical therapy for stone disease.

In emergency settings where concern exists about possible renal failure, the focus of treatment should be on correcting dehydration, treating urinary infections, preventing scarring, identifying patients with a solitary functional kidney, and reducing risks of acute kidney injury from contrast nephrotoxicity, particularly in patients with pre-existing azotaemia (creatinine > 2 mg/dL), diabetes, dehydration, or multiple myeloma.

Adequate intravenous (IV) hydration is essential to minimize the nephrotoxic effects of IV contrast agents.

Most small stones in patients with relatively mild hydronephrosis can be treated with observation and acetaminophen. More serious cases with intractable pain may require drainage with a stent or percutaneous nephrostomy. The internal ureteral stent is usually preferred in these situations because of decreased morbidity.

Acetaminophen can be used in pregnancy for mild-to-moderate pain. Opioid drugs, such as morphine and meperidine, are pregnancy category C medications, which means they can be used but they cross the placental barrier. Opioids can cause respiratory depression in the foetus, therefore, they should not be used near delivery or when other medications are adequate.

A chemical composition analysis of the stone should be performed whenever possible, and information should be provided to motivated patients about possible 24-hour urine testing for long-term nephrolithiasis prophylaxis. This is particularly important in patients with only a single functioning kidney, those with medical risk factors, and children. However, any strongly motivated patients can benefit from a prevention analysis and prophylactic treatment if they are willing to pursue long-term therapy.

The size of the stone is an important predictor of spontaneous passage. A stone less than 4 mm in diameter has an 80% chance of spontaneous passage; this falls to 20% for stones larger than 8 mm in diameter. However, stone passage also depends on the exact shape and location of the stone and the specific anatomy of the upper urinary tract in the particular individual. For example, the presence of ureteropelvic junction (UPJ) obstruction or a ureteral stricture could make passing even very small stones difficult or impossible. Most experienced emergency department (ED) physicians and urologists have observed very large stones passing and some very small stones that do not move.

Aggressive medical therapy has shown promise in increasing the spontaneous stone passage rate and relieving discomfort while minimizing narcotic usage. Aggressive treatment of any proximal urinary infection is important to avoid potentially dangerous pyonephrosis and urosepsis. In these cases, consider percutaneous nephrostomy drainage rather than retrograde endoscopy, especially in very ill patients.

Medical therapy for stone disease takes both short- and long-term forms. The former includes measures to dissolve the stone (possible only with noncalcium stones) or to facilitate stone passage, and the latter includes treatment to prevent further stone formation. Stone prevention should be considered most strongly in patients who have risk factors for increased stone activity, such as the following:

- Stone formation before age 30 years
- Family history of stones

- Multiple stones at presentation
- Residual stones after surgical treatment

In 2016, the American Urological Association/Endourological Society issued general management guidelines for the various presentations of stones that can be managed conservatively. The guidelines state that observation with or without medical expulsive therapy (MET) should be offered to patients with uncomplicated distal ureteral stones that are 10 mm or less in diameter. The guidelines also state that active surveillance can be offered for asymptomatic, non-obstructing caliceal stones.

In the case of pediatric patients with uncomplicated ureteral stones ≤10 mm or asymptomatic non-obstructing renal stones, active surveillance with periodic ultrasonography can be offered. Pregnant patients with ureteral/renal stones with well-controlled symptoms can also be observed.

Indications for hospitalization:

The decision to hospitalize a patient with a stone is usually made based on clinical grounds rather than on any specific finding on a radiograph. Generally, hospitalization for an acute renal colic attack is now officially termed an observation because most patients recover sufficiently to go home within 24 hours. The admission rate for patients with acute renal colic is approximately 20%.

Hospital admission is clearly necessary when any of the following is present:
- Oral analgesics are insufficient to manage the pain.
- Ureteral obstruction from a stone occurs in a solitary or transplanted kidney.
- Ureteral obstruction from a stone occurs in the presence of a urinary tract infection (UTI), fever, sepsis, or pyonephrosis.

Infected hydronephrosis, defined as urinary tract infection (UTI) proximal to an obstructing stone, mandates hospital admission for antibiotics and prompt drainage. Midstream urine culture and sensitivity was a poor predictor of infected hydronephrosis in one series, being positive in only 30% of cases.

Renal ultrasonography or CT may distinguish pyonephrosis from simple hydronephrosis by demonstrating a fluid-fluid level in the renal pelvis (urine on top of purulent debris). In two small studies, ultrasonographic sensitivity for pyonephrosis was found to be 62-67%. CT sensitivity for pyonephrosis has not been reliably determined. The emergency physician must maintain a high index of suspicion.

Relative indications to consider for a possible admission include comorbid conditions (eg, diabetes), dehydration requiring prolonged IV fluid therapy, renal failure, or any immunocompromised state. Patients with complete obstruction, perinephric urine extravasation, a solitary kidney, or pregnancy, and those with a poor social support system, also should be considered for admission, especially if rapid urologic follow-up is not reliably available.

Larger stones (ie, ≥7 mm) that are unlikely to pass spontaneously require some type of surgical procedure. In some cases, hospitalizing a patient with a large stone to facilitate surgical stone intervention is reasonable. However, most patients with acute renal colic can be treated on an ambulatory basis.

About 15-20% of patients require invasive intervention due to stone size, continued obstruction, infection, or intractable pain. Techniques available to the urologist when the stone fails to pass spontaneously include the following

- Stent placement
- Percutaneous nephrostomy
- Extracorporeal shockwave lithotripsy (ESWL)
- Ureteroscopy (URS)
- Percutaneous nephrolithotomy (PCNL) or mini PNCL
- Open nephrostomy - largely supplanted by less-invasive techniques
- Anatrophic nephrolithotomy - increasingly performed using a laparoscopic or robotic approach

Emergency Management of Renal Colic:

Initial treatment of a renal colic patient in the ED starts with obtaining IV access to allow administration of fluid, analgesic, and antiemetic medications. Many of these patients are dehydrated from poor oral intake and vomiting. Although the role of supernormal hydration in the management of renal (ureteral) colic is controversial, patients who are dehydrated or ill need adequate restoration of circulating volume.

After diagnosing renal (ureteral) colic, determine the presence or absence of obstruction or infection. Obstruction in the absence of infection can be initially managed with analgesics and with other medical measures to facilitate passage of the stone. Infection in the absence of obstruction can be initially managed with antimicrobial therapy. In either case, promptly refer the patient to urologist.

If neither obstruction nor infection is present, analgesics and other medical measures to facilitate passage of the stone can be initiated with the expectation that the stone will likely pass from the upper urinary tract if its diameter is smaller than 10 mm (larger stones are more likely to require surgical measures).

If both obstruction and infection are present, emergency decompression of the upper urinary collecting system is required. In addition, immediately consult with urologist for patients whose pain fails to respond to ED management.

ANALGESIC

The ureteral colic management is analgesia, which can be achieved most expediently with parenteral narcotics or nonsteroidal anti-inflammatory drugs (NSAIDs). If oral intake is tolerated, the combination of oral narcotics (eg, codeine, oxycodone, hydrocodone, usually in a combination form with acetaminophen), NSAIDs, and antiemetics, as needed, is a potent outpatient management approach for renal (ureteral) colic.

According to the most recent 2018 Guidelines from the EAU, NSAIDs are now recommended as the first line therapy for pain management over opioids. Recent studies have found them more effective, less likely to require additional pain medications when used, and in the setting of a growing opioid epidemic providers must do their part to minimize patient exposure to the addictive potential of narcotics.

A systematic review and meta-analysis by Hollingsworth et al investigating the role of alpha-blockers in the treatment of ureteric stones addressed pain reduction and a secondary outcome and found that medical expulsive therapy (MET) seemed helpful in reducing pain episodes of patients with acute ureteral colic.

Parenteral narcotics are another mainstay of analgesia for patients with acute renal colic. They work primarily on the central nervous system (CNS) to reduce the perception of pain. They are inexpensive and quite effective. When considering a medication and dosage range, remember that acute renal colic is probably the most painful malady to affect humans. Adverse effects of narcotic analgesics include respiratory depression, sedation, constipation, a potential for addiction, nausea, and vomiting. Respiratory depression is the most concerning adverse effect which caused by a direct effect on the brain stem respiratory centre. This effect is most severe in patients who are elderly, debilitated, or both.

Naloxone (0.4 mg or 1 mL) is a specific narcotic antagonist that can be administered to counteract inadvertent narcotic overdosage or unusual opioid sensitivity. Naloxone has no analgesic properties.

Of the NSAIDs, the only one approved by the US Food and Drug Administration (FDA) for parenteral use is ketorolac. Ketorolac works at the peripheral site of pain production rather than on the CNS. It has been proven in multiple studies to be as effective as opioid analgesics, with fewer adverse effects. The dosage is 30-60 mg IM or 30 mg IV initially followed by 30 mg IV or IM every 6-8 hours. A dose of 15 mg is recommended in patients older than 65 years.

In more severe cases, ketorolac is particularly effective when used together with narcotic analgesics. Oral ketorolac is available in 10-mg pills, but the efficacy of this form in persons with acute renal colic is less clear. Some practitioners use parenteral ketorolac in the hospital but recommend either ibuprofen for pain management in outpatients.

An intranasal ketorolac preparation is available for moderate-to-severe pain and may be particularly useful for outpatient use in patients unable to take oral medication. A maximum of 5 days of ketorolac therapy is recommended.

Chemically, ketorolac is similar to aspirin and may increase the prothrombin time when administered with anticoagulants. Ketorolac can increase methotrexate toxicity and phenytoin levels. It is potentiated by probenecid and should be avoided in patients with peptic ulcer disease, renal failure, or recent gastrointestinal (GI) bleeding.

Antiemetic therapy

Because nausea and vomiting frequently accompany acute renal colic, antiemetics often play a role in renal colic therapy. Several antiemetics have a sedating effect that is often helpful.

Metoclopramide is the only antiemetic that has been specifically studied in the treatment of renal colic. In 2 double-blinded studies, it apparently provided pain relief equivalent to narcotic analgesics in addition to relieving nausea. Its antiemetic effect stems from its dopaminergic receptor blockage in the CNS. It has no anxiolytic activity and is less sedating than other centrally acting dopamine antagonists. The effect of metoclopramide begins within 3 minutes of an IV injection, but it may not take effect for as long as 15 minutes if administered IM. The usual dose in adults is 10 mg IV or IM every 4-6 hours as needed. Metoclopramide is not available as a suppository.

Other medications commonly used as antiemetics include ondansetron, promethazine, prochlorperazine, and hydroxyzine. The author usually recommends antiemetics when patients with renal colic have been vomiting actively or report nausea sufficient to interfere with oral therapy. They also may be useful as anxiolytics in some cases. Ondansetron can provide a useful tool for both emergency room settings as well as at home as it is available in multiple forms including IV, dissolvable tablet, solution and pill form. It has now become the drug of choice for nausea associated with renal colic though is contraindicated in patients with QT prolongation.

Antidiuretic therapy

Several studies have now demonstrated that desmopressin (DDAVP), a potent antidiuretic that is essentially an antidiuretic hormone, can dramatically reduce the pain of acute renal colic in many patients. Though it is not considered standard of care nor has been included in the current AUA or EUA guidelines, it does show potential in certain settings. It acts quickly, has no apparent adverse effects, reduces the need for supplemental analgesic medications, and may be the only immediate therapy necessary for some patients. It is available as a nasal spray (usual dose of 40 mcg, with 10 mcg per spray) and as an IV injection (4 mcg/mL, with 1 mL the usual dose). Generally, only 1 dose is administered.

Animal studies have demonstrated a significant reduction in mean intraureteral pressure after an acute obstruction in subjects administered desmopressin compared with controls. In human studies, approximately 50% of 126 patients tested had complete relief of their acute renal colic pain within 30 minutes after the administration of intranasal desmopressin without any analgesic medication. For patients in whom desmopressin therapy failed, suitable analgesics were administered. No adverse effects from the antidiuretic medication occurred.

Although desmopressin is thought to work by reducing the intraureteral pressure, it may also have some direct relaxing effect on the renal pelvic and ureteral musculature. A central analgesic effect through the release of hypothalamic beta-endorphins has been proposed but remains unproved. Whether this therapy significantly affects eventual stone passage is unknown.

While some of the human studies lack adequate controls and further studies must be conducted, desmopressin therapy currently appears to be a promising alternative or adjunct to analgesic medications in patients with acute renal colic, especially in patients in whom narcotics cannot be used or in whom the pain is unusually resistant to standard medical treatment.

Antibiotic therapy

Antibiotic use in patients with kidney stones remains controversial. Overuse of the more effective agents leaves only highly resistant bacteria, but failure to adequately treat a UTI complicated by an obstructing calculus can result in potentially life-threatening urosepsis and pyonephrosis.

Use antibiotics if a kidney stone or ureteral obstruction has been diagnosed and the patient has clinical evidence of a UTI. Evidence of a possible UTI includes an abnormal finding upon microscopic urinalysis, showing pyuria of 10 WBCs/hpf (or more WBCs than RBCs), bacteriuria, fever, or unexplained leukocytosis. Perform a urine culture in these cases because a culture cannot be performed reliably later should the infection prove resistant to the prescribed antibiotic.

Approximately 3% of patients being treated for renal colic are reported to develop a newly acquired UTI. While case numbers are not high, such an infection can dramatically complicate the clinical outcome for that patient. Base selection of the antibiotic on the patient's presentation, reserving the most effective parenteral antibiotics for patients with frank sepsis or other high-risk characteristics.

The preference for initial medical therapy for pain in patients with acute renal colic is to use IV or IM ketorolac for pain with metoclopramide for nausea. If this therapy is unsuccessful or if the case is deemed more severe, a narcotic such as morphine sulfate or meperidine is added as needed to control pain. An antibiotic is administered if any question of potential infection exists.

Active medical expulsive therapy (MET Therapy)

{NSAIDS, Alpha blockers, Ca channel blocker, Corticosteroides, phosphodiestres inhibitor}

The traditional outpatient treatment approach detailed above has recently been improved with the application of a more aggressive treatment approach known as active medical expulsive therapy (MET). Many randomized trials have confirmed the efficacy of MET in reducing the pain of stone passage, increasing the frequency of stone passage, and reducing the need for surgery.

MET should be considered in any patient with a reasonable probability of stone passage. Given that stones smaller than 3 mm are already associated with an 85% chance of spontaneous passage, MET is probably most useful for stones 3-10 mm in size, though many urologists would argue for the addition of MET with alpha-blockers even with smaller or proximal stones due to the relative in-expense and few side effects for patients undergoing trial of passage if it can potentially avoid need for operative intervention. Overall, MET is associated with a 65% greater likelihood of stone passage with greatest benefits seen with > 5 mm distal stones.

The original rationale for MET was based on the possible causes of failure to spontaneously pass a stone, including ureteral stricture, muscle spasm, local edema, inflammation, and infection. Various common drugs were considered that would potentially benefit these problems, improve spontaneous stone passage, and alleviate renal colic discomfort.

Although NSAIDs have ureteral-relaxing effects and, as such, can be considered a form of MET, they are not generally considered MET.

Corticosteroids have also been considered and tested for MET, though they are not used in current practices due to concerns about unwanted potential side effects, breakthrough pain

The calcium channel blocker Nifedipine is indicated for angina, migraine headaches, Raynaud disease, and hypertension, but it can also reduce muscle spasms in the ureter, which helps reduce pain and facilitate stone passage. Ureteral smooth muscle uses an active calcium pump to produce contractions, so a calcium channel blocker such as Nifedipine would be expected to relax ureteral muscle spasms.

The alpha-blockers, such as terazosin, and the alpha-1 selective blockers, such as tamsulosin, also relax the musculature of the ureter and lower urinary tract, markedly facilitating passage of ureteral stones. Some literature suggests that the alpha-blockers are more effective in this setting than the calcium channel blockers. Currently most practitioners use alpha-blockers preferentially over calcium channel blockers and current guidelines suggest alpha-blockers as the medication of choice for MET.

Multiple prospective randomized controlled studies in the urology literature have demonstrated that patients treated with oral alpha-blockers have an increased rate of spontaneous stone passage and a decreased time to stone passage. The best studied of these is tamsulosin, 0.4 mg administered daily.

A systematic review by Singh et al found that MET using either alpha antagonists or calcium channel blockers augmented the stone expulsion rate for moderately sized distal ureteral stones.

Adverse effects were noted in 4% of those taking alpha antagonists and in 15.2% of those taking calcium channel blockers.

A systematic review by Beach et al found that MET with alpha antagonists for 28 days increased the rate of stone passage, decreased the time to stone passage, and decreased the rates of hospitalization and ureteroscopy, with minimal adverse effects.

Not all data support MET. A randomized study of 77 ED patients with ureterolithiasis found no benefit to a 14-day course of tamsulosin, though the study group was small and the average stone size was 3.6 mm, making spontaneous passage without MET highly likely. Similarly, a prospective, placebo-controlled trial by Pickard et al in 1167 adults with ureteral stones found that neither tamsulosin nor nifedipine decreased the need for further treatment to achieve stone clearance in 4 weeks.

However, Hollingsworth et al propose that the findings of Pickard et al may be largely due to the high rate of spontaneous stone passage in the control group, perhaps because a large proportion of patients had smaller stones. In a systematic review and meta-analysis, these authors concluded that alpha-blockers help facilitate the passage of larger ureteric stones. They recommend considering a course of an alpha-blocker for patients with ureteral colic, unless it is medically contraindicated.

Hollingsworth et al found that overall, passage of larger stones was 57% more likely in patients treated with an alpha-blocker compared with controls (risk ratio 1.57); the likelihood of stone passage increased by 9.8% with every 1 mm increase in stone size. The effect of alpha-blockers was independent of stone location within the ureter. They estimated that four patients would need treatment for one patient to realize benefit from alpha-blockers. Adverse effects associated with alpha-blocker use were relatively infrequent and were not severe.

Additional evidence that alpha-blockers do not expedite the passage of ureteral stones emerged from a randomized clinical trial of 512 adult emergency department patients who presented with renal colic owing to ureteral stones smaller than 9 mm. In this study, the proportion of patients who achieved ureteral stone expulsion by 28 days was 50% with tamsulosin versus 47% with placebo, a nonsignificant difference.

MET with alpha-blockers also appears to improve the results of ESWL as much as the stone fragments resulting from treatment appear to clear the system more effectively.

Analgesic therapy combined with MET dramatically improves the passage of stones, addresses pain, and reduces the need for surgical treatment. Ibuprofen can be substituted for the ketorolac tablets recommended in the original studies. Fewer complications with ibuprofen occur while maintaining efficacy for pain relief. An oral narcotic (eg, oxycodone/acetaminophen) is used as needed to control breakthrough pain.

A typical regimen for this aggressive therapy is as follows:
- 1-2 oral narcotic/acetaminophen tablets every 4 hours as needed for pain

- 600-800 mg ibuprofen every 8 hours

MET with 0.4 mg tamsulosin once daily or 4 mg of terazosin once daily is recommended dosing.

Limit MET to a 10- to 14-day course, as most stones that pass during this regimen do so in that time frame. If outpatient treatment fails, promptly consult urologist.

Future studies may identify a subgroup of patients, such as those with larger stones or history of inability to pass stones that would benefit from MET.

Intravenous hydration

IV hydration in the setting of acute renal colic is controversial. Whereas some authorities believe that IV fluids hasten passage of the stone through the urogenital system, others express concern that additional hydrostatic pressure exacerbates the pain of renal colic. One small study of 43 ED patients found no difference in pain score or rate of stone passage in patients who received 2 L of saline over 2 hours versus those who received 20 mL of saline per hour. [72]

IV hydration should be given to patients with clinical signs of dehydration or to those with a borderline serum creatinine level who must undergo intravenous pyelography (IVP).

Straining urine for stones

Collecting any passed kidney stones is extremely important in the evaluation of a patient with nephrolithiasis for stone-preventive therapy. Yet, in a busy ED, the simple instruction to strain all the urine for stones can be easily overlooked.

Knowing when a stone is going to pass is impossible regardless of its size or location. Even after a stone has passed, residual swelling and spasms can cause continuing discomfort for some time. Be certain that all urine is actually strained for any possible stones. Ideally if patients are seen in the ED, they should be sent home with a strainging device, but in a pinch an aquarium net makes an excellent urinary stone strainer for home use because of its tight nylon weave, convenient handle, and collapsible nature, making it very portable; it easily fits into a pocket or purse.

Surgical Care

In general, stones that are 4 mm in diameter or smaller will probably pass spontaneously, and stones that are larger than 8 mm are unlikely to pass without surgical intervention. With medical expulsive therapy (MET), stones 5-8 mm in size often pass, especially if located in the distal ureter. The larger the stone, the lower the possibility of spontaneous passage (and thus the greater the possibility that surgery will be required), although many other factors determine what happens with a particular stone.

Indications and contraindications

The primary indications for surgical treatment include pain, infection, and obstruction. Infection combined with urinary tract obstruction is an extremely dangerous situation, with significant risk of urosepsis and death, and must be treated emergently in virtually all cases.

The 2016 American Urological Association (AUA)/Endourological Society guidelines provide more specific indications for surgical treatment. The guidelines recommend surgery in the following scenarios:

- Ureteral stones > 10 mm
- Uncomplicated distal ureteral stones ≤10 mm that have not passed after 4-6 weeks of observation, with or without MET
- Symptomatic renal stones in patients without any other etiology for pain
- Pediatric patients with ureteral stones that are unlikely to pass or in whom MET has failed
- Pregnant patients with ureteral or renal stones in whom failed observation has failed

General contraindications to definitive stone manipulation include the following:

- Active, untreated UTI
- Uncorrected bleeding diathesis
- Pregnancy (a relative, but not absolute, contraindication)

Specific contraindications may apply to a given treatment modality. For example, do not perform ESWL if a ureteral obstruction is distal to the calculus or the patient is pregnant.

Surgical options

For an obstructed and infected collecting system secondary to stone disease, virtually no contraindications exist for emergency surgical relief either by ureteral stent placement (a small tube placed endoscopically into the entire length of the ureter from the kidney to the bladder) or by percutaneous nephrostomy (a small tube placed through the skin of the flank directly into the kidney).

Many urologists have a preference for one technique or the other. In general, however, patients who are acutely ill, who have significant medical comorbidities, or who harbor stones that probably cannot be bypassed with ureteral stents undergo percutaneous nephrostomy, whereas others receive ureteral stent placement.

In patients who are floridly septic or hemodynamically unstable, a percutaneous nephrostomy can be a faster and safer way to establish drainage of an infected and obstructed kidney, though airway concerns and other complicating factors such as anticoagulant use or sepsis-associated thrombocytopenia may sway providers towards retrograde stent placement. Ultimately when dealing with seriously ill patients requiring urologic decompression, discussion between urology, anaesthesia and interventional radiology is key to determine the best course of treatment based on positioning and comorbid conditions. Broad-spectrum antibiotics which are then tailored to sensitivities is also paramount whenever a UTI is suspected in conjunction with hydronephrosis or renal colic a septic patient.

The vast majority of symptomatic urinary tract calculi are now treated with non-invasive or minimally invasive techniques. Open surgical excision of a stone from the urinary tract is now limited to isolated atypical cases.

Guidelines are now available to assist the urologist in selecting surgical treatments. The 2005 AUA staghorn calculus guidelines recommend percutaneous nephrostolithotomy as the cornerstone of management; this is consistent with the 2016 AUA/Endourological society and the 2018 EAU guidelines. In the same guidelines, ureteroscopy (URS) is considered the first-line therapy for mid-distal ureteral stones that require intervention, although patients should be offered ESWL if URS is declined.

With regard to renal stones, the guidelines recommend ESWL or URS to symptomatic patients with non–lower pole stones with a total stone burden ≤20 mm or lower pole renal stones ≤10 mm. PCNL is recommended for symptomatic patients with a total renal stone burden >20 mm or lower pole stones >10 mm.

In pediatric patients, URS or ESWL can be offered for ureteral stones that are unlikely to pass or when MET has failed. ESWL or percutaneous nephrostolithotomy can be offered to pediatric patients with a total renal stone burden >20 mm.

Stent placement

Internal ureteral stents form a coil at either end when the stiffening insertion guide wire is removed. One coil forms in the renal pelvis and the other in the bladder. Stents are available in lengths from 20-30 cm and in three widths from 4.6F to 8.5F. Some are designed to soften after placement in the body; others are rather stiff, to resist crushing and obstruction by large stones or external compression with occlusion from an extrinsic tumor or scar tissue.

To select the correct-size stent, estimates can be made based on the height of the patient, or the ureteral length can be measured. This is best performed by means of a retrograde pyelogram. The distance from the tip of the retrograde catheter to the ureteropelvic junction is measured in centimeters with a tape measure. To account for the average magnification effect of the film, 10% of this reading is subtracted. If the result is an odd number, a double-J stent one size longer is used. The most common lengths used are 26 cm in men and 24 cm in women.

The optimal stent width depends on both the relative diameter and course of the ureter and the purpose of the stent. If the patient has a stricture or a tortuous ureter, a stiffer or larger-diameter stent is placed if possible.

When used for stone disease, stents perform several important functions. They virtually guarantee drainage of urine from the kidney into the bladder and bypass any obstruction. This relieves patients of their renal colic pain even if the stone remains. Over time, stents gently dilate the ureter, making ureteroscopy and other endoscopic surgical procedures easier to perform later.

Because they are also quite radiopaque, stents provide a stable landmark when performing ESWL. A landmark is particularly important with small or barely visible stones, especially in the ureter, because the ESWL machine uses radiographic visualization to target the stone. However, routine stent placement should not be performed in patients undergoing ESWL, as there is no difference in stone-free rates with or without stent placement in these patients. [44]

Once large stones are broken up, stents tend to prevent the rapid dumping of large amounts of stone fragments and debris into the ureter (called steinstrasse). The stent forces the fragments to pass slowly, which is more efficient and prevents clogging.

Stents do have drawbacks.

They can become blocked, kinked, dislodged, or infected. A KUB radiograph can be used to determine stent position, while infection is easily diagnosed by urinalysis. A renal sonogram can sometimes be helpful if obstruction is a concern.

Questionable cases can be evaluated further using a radiographic cystogram or an IVP. The cystogram is performed by filling the urinary bladder with diluted contrast media through a Foley catheter under gravity pressure. A stent that is unclogged and functioning normally should show free reflux of contrast from the bladder into the stented renal pelvis.

The major drawback of stents, however, is that they are often quite uncomfortable for patients due to direct bladder irritation, spasm, and reflux. This discomfort can be alleviated to some extent by pain medications, anticholinergics (eg, oxybutynin, tolterodine), alpha-blockers, and topical analgesics (eg, phenazopyridine).

Percutaneous nephrostomy

In some cases, drainage of an obstructed kidney is necessary and stent placement is inadvisable or impossible. In particular, such cases include patients with pyonephrosis who have a UTI or urosepsis exacerbated by an obstructing calculus. In these patients, retrograde endourological procedures such as retrograde pyelography and stent placement may exacerbate infection by pushing infected urinary material into the obstructed renal unit. Percutaneous nephrostomy is useful in such situations. If retrograde stent placement is determined to be more appropriate, attempts to minimize additional pressurization of the collecting system by using minimal contrast and or decompressing prior to contrast administrating should be employed.

Extracorporeal shockwave lithotripsy

ESWL, the least invasive of the surgical methods of stone removal, utilizes high-energy sound waves focused on the stone to shatter it into passable fragments. It is especially suitable for stones that are smaller than 2 cm and lodged in the upper or middle calyx. It is contraindicated in pregnancy, patients with untreatable bleeding disorders, tightly impacted stones, or in cases of ureteral obstruction distal to the stone. In addition, the effectiveness is limited for very hard stones (which tend to be dense on CT scan), cystine stones, and in very large patients.

The patient, under varying degrees of anaesthesia (depending on the type of lithotripter used), is placed on a table or in a gantry that is then brought into contact with the shock head. The deeper the anaesthesia (general endotracheal), the better the results. In addition, evidence is mounting that slower shockwave delivery (60-80 per min) improves the results. Likewise, starting SWL on a lower energy setting with stepwise power (and SWL sequence) ramping has also been advocated in order to achieve vasoconstriction during treatment, which prevents renal injury as well as increase SFR (stone free rates). These are based on findings in some animal studies and a prospective randomized study, but did not find clear evidence of difference in complications or fragmentation size based on use of ramping.

New lithotripters that have two shock heads, which deliver a synchronous or asynchronous pair of shocks (possibly increasing efficacy), have attracted great interest. The shock head delivers shockwaves developed from an electrohydraulic, electromagnetic, or piezoelectric source. The shockwaves are focused on the calculus, and the energy released as the shockwave impacts the stone produces fragmentation. The resulting small fragments pass in the urine.

ESWL is limited somewhat by the size and location of the calculus. A stone larger than 1.5 cm in diameter or one located in the lower section of the kidney is treated less successfully.

Fragmentation still occurs, but the large volume of fragments or their location in a dependent section of the kidney precludes complete passage. In addition, results may not be optimal in large patients, especially if the skin-to-stone distance exceeds 10 cm.

A systematic review found that the majority of studies showed no evidence that ESWL causes long-term adverse effects, including arterial hypertension, diabetes mellitus, kidney dysfunction, or infertility. Nevertheless, a shift seems to be occurring from the use of ESWL to that of ureteroscopy, due to the latter's greater efficacy.

A Cochrane review of seven randomized controlled trials comparing ESWL with ureteroscopy concluded that achievement of a stone-free state occurs more often with ureteroscopy, but ureteroscopy has a higher complication rate and involves a longer hospital stay. A meta-analysis comparing the two approaches showed that although ESWL was just as effective for the management of stones less than 1 cm in the proximal ureter, ureteroscopy otherwise had the following advantages{ref77):

- Higher stone-free rates (92% versus 77%)
- Less frequent need for retreatment (3% versus 21%)
- Greater efficacy in obese patients

Although data have been somewhat conflicting, the EAU and urologic community recommend that MET be used as an adjunct to ESWL to expedite stone passage, increase stone-free rates, and potentially reduce analgesic requirements.

Ureteroscopy

Along with ESWL, ureteroscopic manipulation of a stone (see the image below) is a commonly applied method of stone removal. A small endoscope, which may be rigid, semirigid, or flexible, is passed into the bladder and up the ureter to directly visualize the stone. Normal saline should be used for this procedure, as opposed to sterile water, to prevent electrolyte disturbances and hemolysis.

Ureteroscopy is especially suitable for removal of stones that are 1-2 cm, lodged in the lower calyx or below, cystine stones, and high attenuation ("hard") stones. It is also useful in patients who have multiple small calculi or pre-existing nephrostomy tubes, and following a UTI. The typical patient has acute symptoms caused by a distal ureteral stone, usually measuring 5-8 mm.

Stones smaller than 5 mm in diameter generally are retrieved using a stone basket, whereas tightly impacted stones or those larger than 5 mm are manipulated proximally for ESWL or are fragmented using an endoscopic direct-contact fragmentation device or a holmium laser fiber. Stones can then be retrieved by stone basket and/or allowed to pass spontaneously.

When attempting to achieve a high stone-free rate, a surgeon can take one of two general approaches: 1) complete fragment retrieval via stone basket or 2) exhaustive lithotripsy to allow for residual stones to pass spontaneously. In large studies comparing those two approaches, the former has been associated with higher stone-free rates (up to 100% versus 87%), lower rates of subsequent unplanned emergency department visits, and lower rates of re-hospitalization.

An additional intervention, to prevent migration back into the renal pelvis, is placement of a backstop device proximal to the stone, prior to fragmentation. This has been shown to lead to higher stone-free rates, fewer emergency room visits, and lower hospitalization rates, when compared with cases in which the backstop is not used.

Often, a ureteral stent must be placed after ureteroscopy in order to prevent obstruction from ureteral spasm and edema. Since a ureteral stent is often uncomfortable, many urologists eschew stent placement following ureteroscopy in selected patients. Urologists may omit stent placement in patients who meet all the following criteria·

- No suspected ureteric injury during ureteroscopy
- Absence of ureteral stricture or other anatomical impediments to stone fragment clearance
- Normal contralateral kidney
- No renal function impairment
- No secondary ureteroscopy planned

One of the drawbacks to using rigid or semirigid ureteroscopes for the management of kidney stones is the limited visualization of the entire renal system. This is avoided with the use of a flexible ureteroscope, which allows for visualization of the entire collecting system. The fragility of the fiberoptic instrument is also a concern, with some studies reporting that repairs (often very expensive) were required every 6 to 15 procedures. With regard to the actual stone removal, this procedure requires small stone fragments to allow for retrieval by stone basket. There is also the risk of ureteral injury, which can be reduced with the use of preoperative double-J stenting.

Percutaneous nephrostolithotomy

Percutaneous nephrostolithotomy allows fragmentation and removal of large calculi from the kidney and ureter. Percutaneous procedures have higher morbidity than ESWL and ureteroscopy and so are generally reserved for large and/or complex renal stones and cases in which the other two modalities have failed. Percutaneous nephrostolithotomy is especially useful for stones larger than 2 cm in diameter.

A needle and then a wire, over which is passed a hollow sheath, are inserted directly into the kidney through the skin of the flank. Percutaneous access to the kidney typically involves a sheath with a 1-cm lumen, which will admit relatively large endoscopes with powerful and effective lithotrites that can rapidly fragment and remove large stone volumes. Renal calyces, pelvis, and proximal ureter can be examined and stones extracted with or without prior fragmentation. Normal saline should be used for irrigation, as opposed to sterile water, to prevent electrolyte disturbances and hemolysis.

Stone-free rates for PCNL monotherapy have been shown to be about 56%. As a consequence, multiple sessions of PCNL may be necessary to achieve high stone-free rates. This can result in increased tract-related complications. {ref73) In some cases, a combination of ESWL and a percutaneous technique is necessary to completely remove all stone material from a kidney. This technique, called sandwich therapy, is reserved for staghorn or other complicated stone cases. In such cases, experience has shown that the final procedure should be percutaneous nephrostolithotomy.

Minimally invasive PCNL has been described known as mini-PCNLs, micro-PCNLs or ultra-mini PCNLs. This technique initially was developed in the pediatric population but has become increasingly common in the adult population as well. It involves a 20Fr (0.67 cm) or smaller working sheath for stone manipulation. Stones can then be fragmented with a holmium laser fiber, or pneumatic lithotripter, and removed through the sheath. This method is associated with fewer complications compared with standard PCNL but its efficacy may be limited to stones less than 2 cm; management of larger stones is especially difficult.

Ultra-mini percutaneous nephrolithotomy, which involves use of a small access sheath, has been shown to be safe and effective for the management of renal stones in children. In a study of this technique in 39 pediatric patients (mean age 5.8 ± 4.6 y), complete stone clearance was achieved in 32 patients (82%), increasing to 34 patients (87.1%) 4 weeks post-procedure. No patient required a blood transfusion. Complications occurred in six patients (15.3%).

Anatrophic Nephrolithotomy

Anatrophic nephrolithotomy was classically an open procedure indicated for large staghorn calculi. It involved accessing the kidney through an open approach, identifying the avascular plane of Brodel, which is a relatively avascular plane in the posterior kidney, and then making an incision through this plane and subsequently removing the calculus.

During this procedure the renal artery is clamped, which raises the risk for ischemic injury, as well as reperfusion injury once the procedure is complete. To decrease the risk of those complications, hypothermia of the renal bed is initiated to prevent ischemic injury and intravenous mannitol is given to limit reperfusion injury, due to its ability to attenuate free radical scavengers. This procedure was successful in removing kidney stones, but due to its invasive nature it has been associated with significant morbidity related to the respiratory system (eg, atelectasis, pneumothorax), as well as renal haemorrhage.

A laparoscopic version of this procedure has been developed in more recent years. It involves a three-port access system, similar to other renal procedures. The patient is placed into the flank position and once port access is obtained, the colon is reflected and the hilum is exposed. Intravenous mannitol is given prior to the induction of hypothermia. Methylene blue is then give intravenously, which allows the surgeon to find the avascular plane of Brodel and then mark it using electrocautery.

The renal artery is then clamped and hypothermia is achieved. Hypothermia can be achieved via ice-slush placed in a polythene bag.

Ultrasonography is then used to identify the location of the stones. Next, the incision is made at the previously marked area and the stones are removed.

This technique minimizes the complications encountered in the open approach, while achieving stone-free rates of around 88%. This procedure can be considered for difficult stones that require multiple access tracts throughout the kidney. {ref69)

Unsurprisingly, as robotic-assisted surgery becomes increasingly utilized, it has also been found useful in anatrophic nephrolithotomies. A few small studies have attempted anatrophic nephrolithotomy using a robotic approach. So far it has been shown to be a safe and effective technique that can be used in the removal of large staghorn calculi, with little morbidity. [91, 92]

Open nephrostomy

Open nephrostomy has been used less and less often since the development of ESWL and endoscopic and percutaneous techniques; it now constitutes less than 1% of all interventions. Disadvantages include longer hospitalization, longer convalescence, and increased requirements for blood transfusion.

Invasive therapy during pregnancy

Stone disease in pregnancy poses a particular challenge. In general, conservative management is recommended in the absence of hard indications for surgical intervention such as infection, intractable symptoms, severe hydronephrosis or premature induction of labor.

Regarding imaging modalities, the 2018 EAU guidelines recommend ultrasound as the initial imaging modality of choice. MRI would be a second line choice and low dose CT scans should be saved as a last resort. During pregnancy, radiation may cause teratogenesis or carcinogenesis effects. Teratogenic effects are additive with cumulative doses < 50 mGy considered safe. Gestational age is also important to consider (minimum teratogenic risk prior to 8th week & after 23rd week. Carcinogenesis (dose even < 10 mGy present a risk) and mutagenesis (500-1000 mGy doses are required, far in excess of the doses in common radiographic studies) risks increase with increasing dose but do not require a threshold dose and are not dependent on the gestational age.

Stents and percutaneous nephrostomies unfortunately may be tolerated in pregnant individuals and often require more frequent changes as they have the tendency to rapidly encrust stents.

In a retrospective study of 87 pregnant women who received invasive therapy for proximal ureteral calculi following failure of conservative management, Wang et al found that ureteroscopic holmium laser lithotripsy was more effective and better tolerated postoperatively than cystoscopic double-J stent insertion and percutaneous nephrostom—although all three procedures were effective and safe overall. All 87 women completed a full term of pregnancy without serious obstetric or urologic complications.

Of 64 patients who underwent ureteroscopic lithotripsy, 52 (81.3%) had complete fragmentation of calculi, 9 (14.1%) had retrograde calculi fragments that migrated to the renal pelvis, and 3 had inaccessible calculi due to severe ureteral tortuosity. Of 19 women who underwent cystoscopic double-J stent insertion, 17 (89.5%) were successfully treated; two had guide wire insertion failure (10.5%), were subsequently successfully treated with ureteroscopy, and kept their stents in place until delivery.

Complications of the stent placement included 4 patients who developed urinary tract infections, 12 with stent-induced bladder irritation, and seven with other minor complications. Three of four patients who underwent percutaneous nephrostomy owing to severe hydronephrosis, pyonephrosis, or uncontrolled sepsis were successfully treated. One had extracorporeal shock wave lithotripsy for removal of residual calculi.

Other instruments

Dual wave handheld lithotripters have been described for the use of fragmentation and retrieval of calculi. In the Swiss Lithoclast, for example, one probe is a pneumatic lithotripter and the other is an ultrasonic lithotripter. The pneumatic component is used to break up large stones and the ultrasound component contains a suction device, which is used for stone retrieval. It has been shown to be a safe and quick technique for bladder calculi.

Another instrument introduced in recent years is the StoneBreaker, which is a novel handheld pneumatic lithotripter powered by compressed carbon dioxide. The StoneBreaker has been shown to be more effective than the Swiss LIthoclast in the management of staghorn calculi.

Medical Therapy for Stone Disease

Dissolution of calculi

Urinary calculi composed predominantly of calcium cannot be dissolved with current medical therapy; however, medical therapy is important in the long-term chemoprophylaxis of further calculus growth or formation.

Uric acid and cystine calculi can be dissolved with medical therapy. Patients with uric acid stones who do not require urgent surgical intervention for reasons of pain, obstruction, or infection can often have their stones dissolved with alkalization of the urine. Sodium bicarbonate can be used as the alkalizing agent, but potassium citrate is usually preferred because of the availability of slow-release tablets and the avoidance of a high sodium load. In patients with recurrent calcium stones and low urinary citrate levels, potassium citrate therapy should be offered. For patients with obstructing uric acid stones in the collecting system that do not require surgical intervention, a combination of alkalinization with tamsulosin can increase the frequency of spontaneous passage of distal ureteral uric acid stones as shown in one RCT for stones > 5 mm. [97]

The dosage of the alkalizing agent should be adjusted to maintain the urinary pH between 6.5 and 7.0. Urinary pH of more than 7.5 should be avoided because of the potential deposition of calcium phosphate around the uric acid calculus, which would make it undissolvable. Both uric acid and cystine calculi form in acidic environments.

Even very large uric acid calculi can be dissolved in patients who comply with therapy. Roughly 1 cm per month dissolution can be achieved. Practical ability to alkalinize the urine significantly limits the ability to dissolve cystine calculi.

Chemoprophylaxis

Prophylactic therapy might include limitation of dietary components, addition of stone-formation inhibitors or intestinal calcium binders, and, most importantly, augmentation of fluid intake. (See Dietary Measures and Prevention of Nephrolithiasis.) Besides advising patients to avoid excessive salt and protein intake and to increase fluid intake, base medical therapy for long-term chemoprophylaxis of urinary calculi on the results of a 24-hour urinalysis for chemical constituents.

In patients with high urine calcium levels and recurrent calcium stones, thiazide diuretics are recommended. In patients with recurrent calcium stones and low or relatively low urinary citrate, potassium citrate should be offered. If a patient suffers from recurrent calcium stones but metabolic abnormalities are absent or controlled with treatment, thiazides, potassium citrate, or both should be offered. [98]

Chemoprophylaxis of uric acid and cystine calculi consists primarily of long-term alkalinization of urine with potassium citrate. If hyperuricosuria or hyperuricemia is documented in patients with pure uric acid stones (present in only a relative minority), allopurinol (300 mg qd) is recommended because it reduces uric acid excretion. Allopurinol should also be offered to patients with recurrent calcium oxalate stones who have hyperuricosuria and normal urinary calcium levels. [98]

Pharmaceuticals that can bind free cystine in the urine (eg, D-penicillamine, 2-alpha-mercaptopropionyl-glycine) help reduce stone formation in cystinuria. Therapy should also include long-term urinary alkalinization and aggressive fluid intake.

Dietary Measures

In almost all patients in whom stones form, an increase in fluid intake and, therefore, an increase in urine output is recommended. This is likely the single most important aspect of stone prophylaxis. Patients with recurrent nephrolithiasis traditionally have been instructed to drink 8 glasses of fluid daily to maintain adequate hydration and decrease chance of urinary supersaturation with stone-forming salts. The goal is a total urine volume in 24 hours in excess of 2.5 liters.

The only other general dietary guidelines are to avoid excessive salt and protein intake. Moderation of calcium and oxalate intake is also reasonable, but great care must be taken not to indiscriminantly instruct the patient to reduce calcium intake. Patients with calcium stones and relatively low urinary citrate should increase their intake of fruits and vegetables.

Dietary calcium should not be restricted beyond normal unless specifically indicated on the basis of on 24-hour urinalysis findings. Urinary calcium levels are normal in many patients with calcium stones. Reducing dietary calcium in these patients may actually worsen their stone disease, because more oxalate is absorbed from the GI tract in the absence of sufficient intestinal calcium to bind with it. This results in a net increase in oxalate absorption and hyperoxaluria, which tends to increase new kidney stone formation in patients with calcium oxalate calculi.

An empiric restriction of dietary calcium may also adversely affect bone mineralization and may have osteoporosis implications, especially in women. This practice should be condemned unless indicated based on a metabolic evaluation.

As a rule, dietary calcium should be restricted to 1000-1200 mg/d in patients with diet-responsive hypercalciuria who form calcium stones. This is roughly equivalent to a single high-calcium or dairy meal per day.

Prevention of Nephrolithiasis

The most common causes of kidney stones are hypercalciuria, hyperuricosuria, hyperoxaluria, hypocitraturia, and low urinary volume. Each of these major factors can be measured easily with a 24-hour urine sample using one of several commercial laboratory packages now available. Kidney stone preventive therapy consists of dietary adjustments, nutritional supplements, medications, or combinations of these.

Strongly encourage patients who have a stone at a young age (ie, < 25 y), multiple recurrences, a solitary functioning kidney, or a history of prior kidney stone surgery to obtain a 24-hour urine collection for stone prevention analysis, especially if they are motivated to comply with a long-term stone prevention program. These 24-hour urine collection kits can be obtained from a number of commercial medical laboratories.

Consultations

Consultation with urologist is required when immediate ED management of renal (ureteral) colic fails. Referral to urologist is necessary for all stones that prove refractory to outpatient management or that fail to pass spontaneously.

Consult a urologist immediately in cases of ureterolithiasis with proximal UTI. Infected hydronephrosis is a true urologic emergency and requires hospital admission, IV fluids, IV antibiotics, and immediate drainage of the infected hydronephrosis via percutaneous nephrostomy or ureteral stent placement.

Urologic consultation is also appropriate in patients with unusually large stones, high-risk medical conditions, inability to tolerate oral fluids and medications, unrelenting pain, renal failure, renal transplant, a solitary functioning kidney, or a history of prior stones that required invasive intervention.

Patients who are pregnant require a consultation with an obstetrician-gynecologist, and those with a history of severe cardiac disease or congestive heart failure may benefit from involvement of an internal medicine specialist or cardiologist.

Patients with strong motivation to prevent all future stones, those with multiple recurrences or single functioning kidneys, and all children younger than 16 years with nephrolithiasis should be referred to a specialist in nephrolithiasis prevention. A medical expert in metabolic stone prevention testing, interpretation, and prophylactic therapy is available in most communities.

Long-Term Monitoring

Patients who do not meet admission criteria may be discharged from the ED in anticipation that the stone will pass spontaneously at home. Arrangements should be made for follow-up with a urologist in 2-3 days. Patients should be told to return immediately for fever, uncontrolled pain, or inability to tolerate oral intake which can lead to dehydration. Patients should be discharged with a urine strainer and encouraged to submit any recovered calculi to a urologist for chemical analysis.

Follow-up for patients with first-time incidence of stones should consist of stone analysis and abbreviated metabolic evaluation to rule out hyperparathyroidism, renal tubular acidosis, and chronic infection with urea-splitting bacteria.

Patients with recurrent ureterolithiasis should undergo a more thorough metabolic evaluation. Patients with recurrent stones who undergo thorough metabolic evaluation and specific therapy enjoy a remission rate in excess of 80% and can decrease the rate of stone formation by 90%. A stone chemical analysis together with serum and appropriate 24-hour urine metabolic tests can identify the etiology in more than 95% of patients.

A typical 24-hour urine determination should include urinary volume, pH, specific gravity, calcium, citrate, magnesium, oxalate, phosphate, and uric acid. Most common findings are hypercalciuria, hyperuricosuria, hyperoxaluria, hypocitraturia, and low urinary volume.

Postsurgical follow-up

After surgical treatment of urinary tract calculi, the major issues include infection, ureteral obstruction, and hemorrhage. The postoperative course of minimally invasive stone-removal modalities is generally characterized by short-lived discomfort easily managed with oral medications. Continued or severe pain should prompt evaluation for complications. Repeat urine cultures and imaging studies should be performed to assess for ureteral obstruction and perforation, and the degree of circulating blood volume should be evaluated for ongoing hemorrhage.

The importance of office follow-up and examination should be stressed with patients. Though EAU and AUA guidelines have not provided a consensus statement regarding timing or modality specifics for follow-up imaging, it is recommended that some imaging modality be completed in the post-operative setting. Undiagnosed residual stone fragments and silent hydronephrosis pose potential threats in post-operative settings. The most recent 2018 EAU guideline suggests follow up imaging around one month. [1]

Once postoperative complications have been excluded and the patient is clinically healthy, standard radiographic follow-up care includes abdominal radiography or ultrasound every 6-12 months. Imaging is often performed in conjunction with metabolic chemoprophylaxis. Above and beyond this, additional imaging is often unnecessary in a patient with a previous radiopaque stone who has no further symptoms. Imaging that includes assessment of renal drainage (eg, IVP, ultrasonography, CT scanning) is usually indicated in the following cases:

- Stones with unusual characteristics
- Difficult or complicated procedures
- Patients with unusual symptoms

Ongoing medical therapy

If a patient older than 40 years has formed a single stone that passed spontaneously or was easily treated, follow-up care for recurrent stones may be unnecessary. Such patients are at a reasonably low risk for recurrence if they maintain adequate fluid intake. In other patients, whether or not they have elected directed metabolic therapy, routine follow-up care consists of plain abdominal radiography (or renal ultrasonography in the case of radiolucent stones) every 6-12 months.

If medical therapy is instituted, a 24-hour urinalysis 3 months after starting any new therapy should be performed to assess the degree of patient compliance and the adequacy of the metabolic response. Checking all possible metabolic parameters—not just the previously abnormal ones—is necessary because of the possibility of new problems arising as a result of the new therapy. Once a stable regimen has been established, annual 24-hour urinalyses are adequate.